Dual Energy CT in Oncology

Carlo N. De Cecco • Andrea Laghi
U. Joseph Schoepf • Felix G. Meinel

Editors

Dual Energy CT
in Oncology

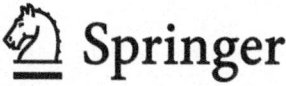 Springer

Editors
Carlo N. De Cecco
Medical University of South Carolina
Charleston, SC
USA

Andrea Laghi
Sapienza University of Rome
Rome
Italy

U. Joseph Schoepf
Medical University of South Carolina
Charleston, SC
USA

Felix G. Meinel
Ludwig-Maximilians-University Hospital
Munich
Germany

ISBN 978-3-319-36084-3   ISBN 978-3-319-19563-6   (eBook)
DOI 10.1007/978-3-319-19563-6

Springer Cham Heidelberg New York Dordrecht London
© Springer International Publishing Switzerland 2015
Softcover reprint of the hardcover 1st edition 2015

Printed on acid-free paper

Springer International Publishing AG Switzerland is part of Springer Science+Business Media
(www.springer.com)

Preface

Dual energy CT is an innovative imaging technique which has recently entered clinical practice. Despite its recent introduction, the number of CT scanners with dual energy capabilities is growing rapidly, and new clinical applications are already available or under investigation. With rising clinical interest and an established base of scanner technology, DECT will increasingly figure into clinical routine as radiologists further integrate DECT in their daily practice.

As detailed in this book, DECT acquisition allows the simultaneous generation of multiple datasets including iodine density map, virtual monochromatic or virtual unenhanced images, and elemental decomposition analyses which aid the radiologist in addressing various diagnostic problems using a multiparametric approach. When routinely applied, these applications of DECT may be particularly useful in oncologic imaging, providing clear advantages in tumor detection, lesion characterization, and evaluation of response to therapy.

A growing body of evidence demonstrating the value of DECT applications in different oncological fields is rapidly accumulating, and we strongly believe that DECT represents a significant step forward in the continued quest to improve our diagnostic capabilities.

This book is intended for radiologists as well as specialists who are currently using DECT or intend to start using this new fascinating diagnostic technique in their clinical practice. The first section of the book outlines the technical basis of dual energy imaging, investigating the different approaches present in the current market and describing existing post-processing techniques. The second section focuses on the clinical use and interpretation of DECT and its impact on clinical decision making in a variety of oncological settings, including tumors of the head and neck, lung, liver, pancreas, gastrointestinal system, kidney, and musculoskeletal system.

It is our sincere hope that readers will find this book useful in their clinical practice and that our efforts will contribute to the growing investigation and application of this exciting technique.

Charleston, SC, USA   Carlo N. De Cecco
Rome, Italy   Andrea Laghi
Charleston, SC, USA   U. Joseph Schoepf
Munich, Germany   Felix G. Meinel
May 2015

Contents

Dual Energy CT: Basic Principles

Luca Saba, Michele Porcu, Bernhard Schmidt,
and Thomas Flohr

1.1 Introduction

Computed tomography (CT), since its introduction in the 1970s, has not only revolutionized radiology, but made all diagnostic algorithms faster and more accurate: for example, the presence of a subdural hematoma in a trauma patient before the invention of CT could be just suspected after an accurate neurological examination and by the presence of a fracture of the skull on a conventional x-ray. Nowadays, a CT scan performed in few seconds clearly shows the presence and the characteristics of the lesion.

Dual Energy Computed Tomography (DECT) is a new promising technology, already available in clinical practice, which can offer new advantages for radiologists and clinicians, thanks to its intrinsic ability to characterize tissue composition.

1.2 Basic Principles of Single Energy Computed Tomography

Single energy CT (SECT) scanners provide cross-sectional images of the human body through the use of x-rays. The measurement system of a SECT comprises an x-ray tube and an opposing detection system (DS) which rotate around the patient. The DS consists of an array of small detectors. Typically, 700–900 individual

L. Saba • M. Porcu
Department of Radiology, Azienda Ospedaliero Universitaria (A.O.U.),
Via Tola 7, 09128 Cagliari, Italy
e-mail: lucasabamd@gmail.com

B. Schmidt • T. Flohr (✉)
Computed Tomography, Siemens Healthcare, Siemensstr. 1, 91301 Forchheim, Germany
e-mail: thomas.flohr@siemens.com

© Springer International Publishing Switzerland 2015
C.N. De Cecco et al. (eds.), *Dual Energy CT in Oncology*,
DOI 10.1007/978-3-319-19563-6_1

detector elements are placed next to each other to cover the scan field of view (SFOV) of 50 cm diameter. The detectors record the intensities of the x-rays after passing through the patient and convert them into electrical currents that are digitized by the Data Acquisition System (DAS). During a CT scan, about 700–900 measurement values are recorded at about 1000 angular positions per rotation. These so-called CT raw data undergo mathematical operations in the image reconstruction process to transform them into a CT image.

When crossing the human body, the x-rays interact with the molecules that constitute the human tissues. They are attenuated and reach the DS with a lower intensity (I) than the primary intensity (I_0), according to Eq. 1.1:

$$I = I_0 e^{-\int_0^L \mu(x,y,z)ds} \tag{1.1}$$

Here μ is the linear attenuation coefficient of the x-rays at point (x, y, z), L is the thickness of the tissue crossed by the x-ray beam, and s is the coordinate along the path of the x-ray beam.

According to Eq. 1.2 (derived from Eq. 1.1),

$$\int_0^L \mu(x,y,z)ds = -\ln\left(\frac{I}{I_0}\right) \tag{1.2}$$

is the line integral of the x-ray attenuation coefficient μ. The line integrals, recorded at different angular position of the measurement system, are the basic measurement parameters in CT. In the image reconstruction process, the local x-ray attenuation coefficients μ are extracted and stored in the image matrix constituted by voxels (pixels in the CT image) with specific coordinates (x, y, z).

The value μ is characteristic for every voxel of the image matrix, and in SECT it is converted to the Hounsfield Units (HU) value scale according Eq. 1.3:

$$CT\,number(HU) = 1000 \times \frac{\mu(x,y,z) - \mu_{(water)}}{\mu_{(water)}} \tag{1.3}$$

Here, $\mu_{(water)}$ is the x-ray attenuation coefficient of water.

In a single energy CT scan, the technician can adjust different scan parameters in order to obtain an optimal examination, in particular modifying the intensity and the energy of the x-rays.

The intensity of the x-rays depends directly on the tube current of the x-ray tube.

The energy of the x-rays is directly proportional to the differential in potential (ΔV) between the cathode and the anode of the x-ray tube (or in other words it depends on the applied tube voltage). The value of ΔV is expressed in kV.

- For *high tube voltage*, the x-ray beam will be absorbed less in the human body and have higher penetration, and a relatively large amount of x-ray quanta will reach the DS. At a given primary x-ray intensity I_0, image noise will be low. On the other hand, the contrast resolution of the image will be reduced, in particular for CT examinations obtained after intravenous administration of iodine-based contrast agent.

- For *low tube voltage*, the x-rays beam will show higher absorption and less penetration in the human body. The x-rays will interact more with the structures of the human body, and at a given primary x-ray intensity I_0, a smaller amount of x-ray quanta will reach the DS, increasing image noise on the one hand but improving the contrast resolution of the image on the other.

1.3   X-Ray Spectrum and K-Shell Binding Energy

The generation of x-rays in the x-ray tube is a probabilistic process that produces a spectrum of x-rays at different energies. The energy of the x-rays is expressed in keV. The maximum energy of the x-ray spectrum corresponds to the applied tube voltage, its mean energy is directly proportional to it. The spectrum is superimposed by peaks characteristic for the anode material.

A typical x-ray spectrum is shown in Fig. 1.1, and the shape of the curve (and so the x-ray intensity at a certain energy) changes with the applied tube voltage.

In clinical practice, x-ray tube voltages between 70 and 140 kV are used in CT. For these values, the energy spectrum comprises a range between 30 and 140 keV [1], with a *mean energy* of about 52 keV for 80 kV tube voltage and 69 keV for 140 kV tube voltage (directly behind the bowtie filter and depending on the prefiltration of the spectrum) [2].

In this energy range, there are basically two interaction mechanisms of the x-rays with the atoms and molecules of the human body [1, 3, 4]:

- *Compton scattering*: When an x-ray photon hits an electron of the external orbitals (or shells) having a low binding energy, it loses a part of its energy and its trajectory is deflected before reaching the DS, while the electron is knocked out from its orbital. Compton scattering is responsible for a loss of contrast resolution of the images [3]. It predominates in areas of the human body rich in atoms with low atomic number (see below) [5], and it mainly depends on the density of the material [6].
- *Photoelectric absorption*: When an x-ray photon hits an electron of the innermost orbital (noted as K-shell), it loses all its energy, the electron is knocked out from its orbital, and the x-ray photon does not reach the DS [3]. This phenomenon prevails in tissues rich in atoms with high atomic number (see below) [5], and it depends strongly on the x-ray energy and on the atomic number of the material.

The K-shell binding energy is directly proportioned to the atomic number of the respective elements [3]. Elements such as hydrogen ($Z=1$), carbon ($Z=6$), nitrogen ($Z=7$) and oxygen ($Z=8$) have a small K-shell binding energy between 0.01 and

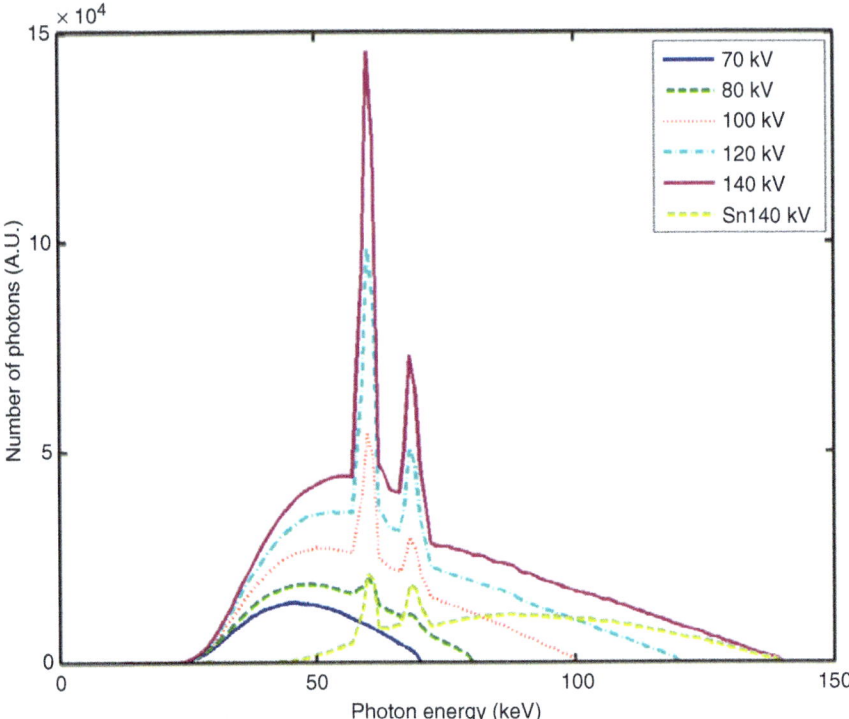

Fig. 1.1 Typical x-ray spectra used in medical CT. The spectra at 70, 80, 100, 120, and 140 kV are obtained after standard pre-filtration. Their mean energies range between 47 and 69 keV. The Sn 140 kV spectrum is obtained after pre-filtration with 0.4 mm Sn (tin) to remove lower energy x-ray quanta and shift the mean energy of the spectrum to higher values

0.53 keV, in comparison with calcium ($Z = 20$, K-shell binding energy 4.0 keV) and iodine ($Z = 53$, K-shell binding energy 33.2 keV) [2, 3].

The probability of photoelectric absorption is larger if the x-ray energy is similar to the K-shell binding energy [3, 5] and for low values of the x-ray tube voltage [4]. For x-ray energies just above the K-shell binding energy, there is a sudden increase in attenuation, because then the x-ray quantum will lose all its energy to the K-shell electron and will no longer reach the DS. This increase in x-ray attenuation translates into an increase in the HU values of the image [3].

1.4 From Single Energy Computed Tomography to Dual Energy Computed Tomography

In SECT, the scan is performed with a specific x-ray tube voltage according to the characteristics of the patient and the examination type.

For different values of the x-ray tube voltage, the energy spectrum of the x-rays will be different, and x-ray quanta will interact with matter in different ways:

- For tissues rich in elements with high atomic number (for example calcium and the iodine of the contrast medium), the mean energy of the x-ray spectrum will be closer to the K-shell binding energy if low tube voltages are chosen. The photoelectric effect predominates, and the HU values will be higher compared with scans at high tube voltage [3–5].
- For tissues mainly containing elements with low atomic number, such as hydrogen, carbon, nitrogen, and oxygen (for example fat, or muscles), the K-shell binding energy values are very low and do not differ significantly (from 0.01 keV for hydrogen to 0.53 keV for oxygen). As a consequence, there will be no great difference in attenuation of the x-rays when high or low tube voltages are used [4].

To summarize, the x-ray attenuation μ mainly depends on three parameters:

- The elements that constitute the region of interest
- The density of the region of interest
- The x-ray spectrum for the specific tube voltage ΔV

The x-ray attenuation μ at a specific x-ray energy E can be decomposed into attenuation caused by Compton scattering and attenuation caused by the photoelectric effect, see Eq. 1.4 [7]:

$$\mu_{(x,y,z)}(E) = \mu_{Compton}(E) + \mu_{photoelectric}(E) \tag{1.4}$$

Here $\mu_{(x,y,z)}(E)$ is the x-ray attenuation at a specific point (x, y, z).

Using a single x-ray spectrum, two different object regions can have the same attenuation μ even if they differ in chemical composition and material density. As an example, calcified plaques in a vessel can often not be differentiated from the surrounding lumen in the presence of iodinated contrast agent.

Using two different x-ray spectra with two different mean energies E_1 and E_2 in a dual energy CT (DECT) scan can help characterize the material composition of the tissues, because Eq. 1.4 can then be resolved for both $\mu_{Compton}(E)$ and $\mu_{photoelectric}(E)$.

Moreover, $\mu_{(x,y,z)}(E)$ of any material can be decomposed into a linear combination of the attenuation of two base materials 1 and 2, which differ in their photoelectric and Compton characteristics. The relative contributions of these two base materials to each voxel of interest can be determined by measurements with two different spectra [1–5].

1.5 Dual Energy CT Scanners Available in Clinical Practice

In clinical practice, there are several methods to acquire DECT data [2]. Most commonly, two different x-ray spectra are used in combination with standard CT detectors. In commercially available solutions, a variety of different techniques has been introduced:

- Performing two subsequent scans with different x-ray tube voltages with a single source CT scanner
- Rapidly switching the x-ray tube voltage during the scan
- Introducing a split filter into the tube collimator housing of a single source CT scanner
- Using dual source CT systems
- Another approach uses a single x-ray spectrum in combination with an energy-sensitive detector (dual layer detector).

CT systems with photon counting detectors are still in research state. So far, only pre-clinical prototypes have been available. CT systems with photon counting detectors will therefore not be discussed in detail here.

1.5.1 Scans with Different X-Ray Tube Voltages with a Single Source CT Scanner

This technique has been developed to acquire dual energy data with single source CT scanners without further system modification, such as rapid kV-switching, use of dual layer detectors or split filters in the tube collimator housing [3]. It requires the execution of two consecutive CT scans at different x-ray tube voltages, either in sequential (axial) or spiral (helical) mode. Most commonly, 80 and 140 kV are used, because these are typically the lowest and highest kV settings of a CT x-ray tube which provide best spectral separation, see Fig. 1.2.

Because of the long time delay between the different acquisitions, examinations with administration of contrast agent are difficult, at least in early arterial phases when the contrast density changes rapidly [2, 3].

There are different commercial realizations of this DE acquisition principle [2, 3]:

- In the Volume Dual Energy approach (*GE Healthcare, Milwaukee, Wis, USA*), alternating sequential scans of the same body region are performed at different x-ray tube voltages [3]. Because of the relatively long delay between the sequential acquisitions and the long total scanning time (e.g., 20 s for a single-phase scan of the liver), the Volume Dual Energy technique has been evaluated in prototypes, but never introduced into the market [3].
- With increasing z-coverage of the detectors (the z-axis is the patient's longitudinal direction) and faster gantry rotation time, larger anatomical areas can be covered with one sequential scan, and the delay between subsequent acquisitions at different x-ray tube voltages becomes shorter. Two different vendors offer single source CT scanners with 16 cm detector z-coverage (*Aquilion One; Toshiba, Tochigi, Japan* and *Revolution, GE Healthcare, Milwaukee, Wis, USA*), capable of scanning organs such as the heart without table movement. Both systems acquire dual energy data by performing fast sequential scans with two different tube voltages at gantry rotation times of 0.27 s or 0.28 s [5].
- Another commercially available technical realization relies on two subsequent spiral (helical) scans of the same body region (*Somatom Definition Edge; Siemens Healthcare, Forchheim, Germany*), the first one at 80 kV and the second

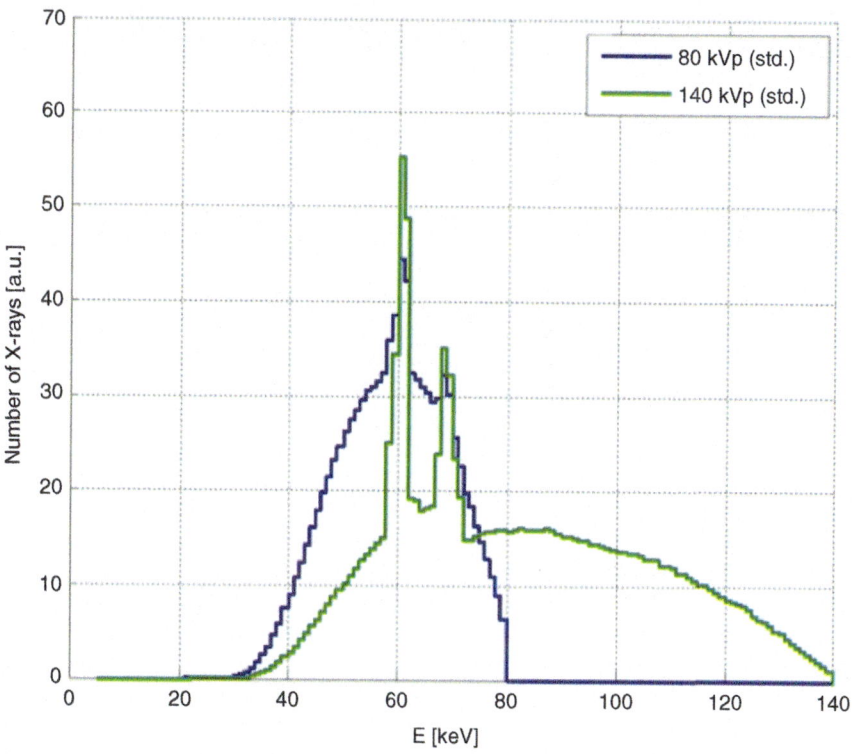

Fig. 1.2 Standard 80 and 140 kV spectra (normalized to equal intensity) used to acquire DE data at two different x-ray tube voltages

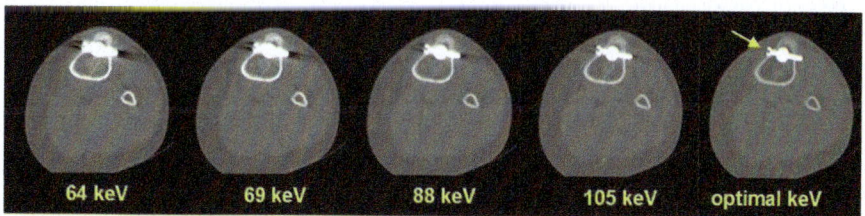

Fig. 1.3 Clinical example demonstrating the use of pseudo mono-energetic images to reduce metal artifacts. The DE scan data were obtained using two consecutive spiral scans at 80 and 140 kV

one at 140 kV. As in standard CT examinations, radiation dose to the patient can be optimized by anatomical tube current modulation [3]. Because of the relatively long time delay between the two spiral scans, the use of this technique is indicated for nondynamic examinations that do not require the administration of contrast agent, such as characterization of kidney stones or the examination of tophaceous lesions in patients with gout [3], or for the calculation of mono-energetic images to reduce metal artifacts at a metal-specific high energy. Figure 1.3 shows a clinical example.

Fig. 1.4 Schematic
illustration of rapid
kV-switching between
80 and 140 kV tube
voltage. Note that two
or more low kV
projections are acquired
for each high kV
projection to balance
radiation dose

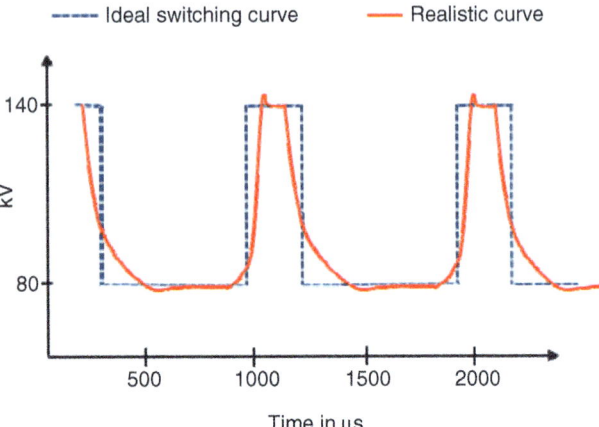

1.5.2 Rapid Switching of the X-Ray Tube Voltage During the Scan

In a more refined approach, the kV-setting of the x-ray tube is rapidly switched between consecutive projections of the same axial or spiral scan. The *Discovery 750HD* scanner (*GE Healthcare, Milwaukee, Wis, USA*) is equipped with an x-ray tube and a corresponding generator capable of switching the ΔV peak values from 80 to 140 kV and vice versa in about 0.25 ms during scan data acquisition [1–5] (Fig. 1.4). According to the manufacturer, the CT scanner uses a detection system (*Gemstone detector; GE Healthcare, Milwaukee, Wis*) characterized by a faster emission of light and shorter afterglow time if compared with standard scintillation detectors [3, 5, 7].

One advantage of rapid kV-switching is the almost simultaneous acquisition of low-energy and high-energy projections with a time delay of less than 0.5 ms, which prevents registration problems due to organ motion or contrast agent dynamics. Dual energy scan data are acquired in the full SFOV of 50 cm diameter [3, 5].

As a downside, fast switching of the x-ray tube current simultaneously to the fast switching of the x-ray tube voltage is technically not possible, and at equal x-ray tube current the x-ray flux at 80 kV is much lower than at 140 kV [2, 3, 5]. To balance the radiation dose of the low kV and the high kV data, two or more low kV projections are acquired for every single high kV projection, see Fig. 1.4. As a consequence, however, the total number of high kV projections during one rotation is reduced, resulting in potential sampling problems and limiting the maximum achievable spatial resolution. As of today, optimizing the radiation dose to the patient by using anatomical dose modulation is not possible. The potentially increased overall radiation dose can at least partially be reduced by combining DE data acquisition with the use of iterative reconstruction (*Adaptive Statistical Iterative Reconstruction [ASIR]; GE Healthcare, Milwaukee, Wis*) [2, 3, 5]. As another disadvantage, spectral separation cannot be improved by introducing separate

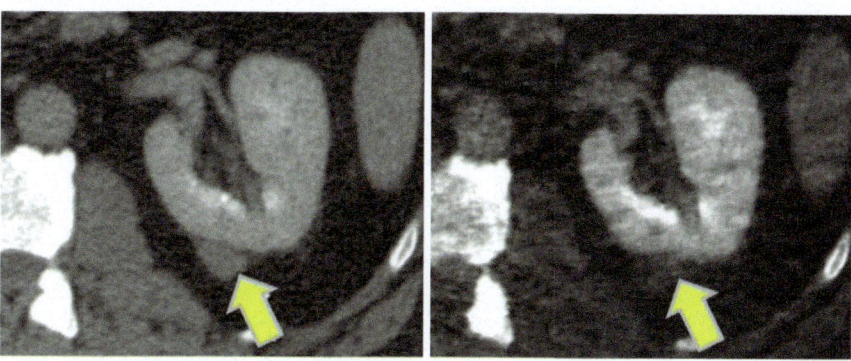

Fig. 1.5 Clinical example of DE data acquisition by means of rapid kV-switching. *Left*: Pseudo mono-energetic image at 75 keV reveals a lesion with attenuation 57 HU (*arrow*). *Right*: Iodine density map indicates a lack of iodine enhancement (*arrow*), which is characteristic for a cyst (From [8])

pre-filtration of the low kV and the high kV beam (see below). As a practical clinical limitation, the manufacturer provides only images from the 140 kV data set and not from the 80 kV data set [3]. Figure 1.5 shows a clinical example.

1.5.3   Use of a Split Filter in the Tube Collimator Housing

Recently, a new method was introduced to acquire DECT data with a single source CT system without kV-switching, but with better temporal registration than by performing two separate consecutive sequential or spiral scans of the examination volume of interest.

In the *Twin Beam* dual energy approach (*Somatom Definition Edge, Siemens Healthcare, Forchheim, Germany*), two different pre-filters in the tube collimator housing are used to split the x-ray beam in the z-axis direction (the z-axis is the patient's longitudinal direction), see Fig. 1.6.

The x-ray tube is operated at 120 kV tube voltage. One-half of the multi-slice detector in the z-axis direction is illuminated by an x-ray beam pre-filtered with 0.6 mm tin – compared to the standard 120 kV spectrum, the mean energy of this pre-filtered spectrum is shifted to higher energies, see Fig. 1.7. The other half of the detector in the z-axis direction is pre-filtered with a thin gold filter – because of the K-edge of gold at 80.7 keV, the mean energy of this spectrum is shifted to somewhat lower energies, see Fig. 1.7. The total attenuation of the pre-filters is adjusted such as to balance the radiation dose of the low-energy and the high-energy beam. The CT system is operated in a spiral (helical) scan mode at fast gantry rotation speed (0.28 s) and with a maximum spiral pitch of 0.75 (referring to the full z-width of the detector). Then, each half of the detector acquires a complete spiral data set, and both low-energy and high-energy images can be reconstructed at any z-position.

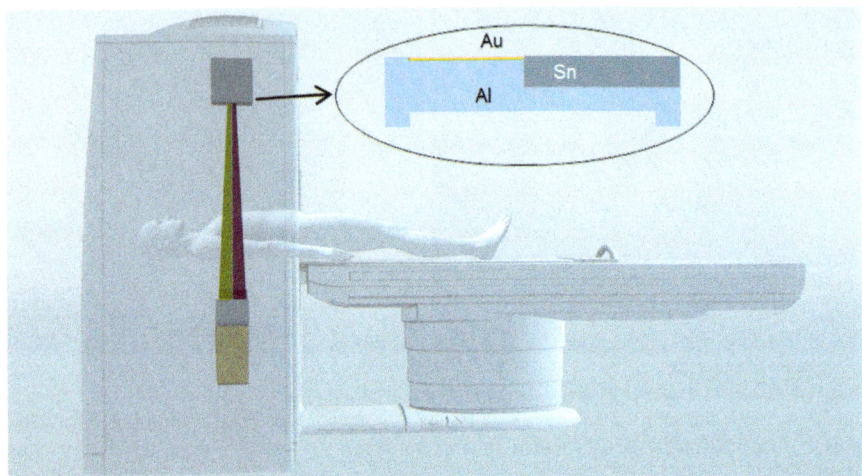

Fig. 1.6 Principle of a DE acquisition technique that makes use of a split filter in the tube collimator housing to split the x-ray beam in the patient's longitudinal direction into a low-energy and a high-energy beam

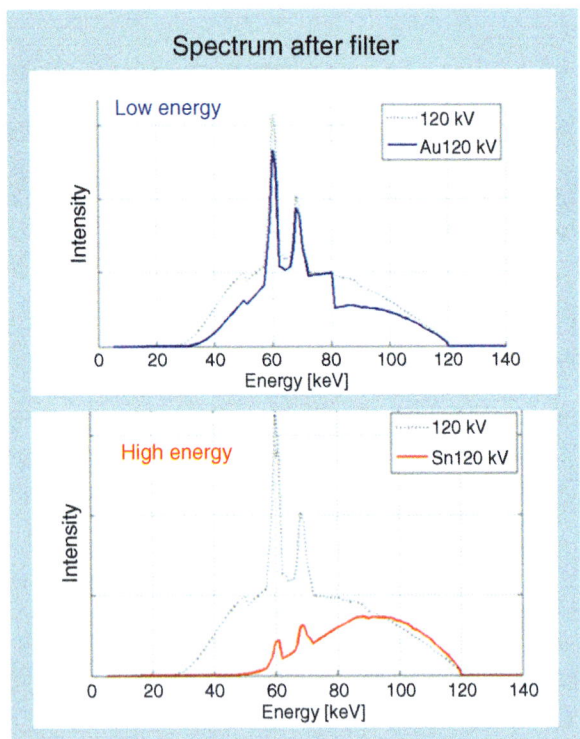

Fig. 1.7 Low-energy and high-energy spectra after pre-filtration of a 120 kV spectrum with Au (*top*) and tin (*bottom*)

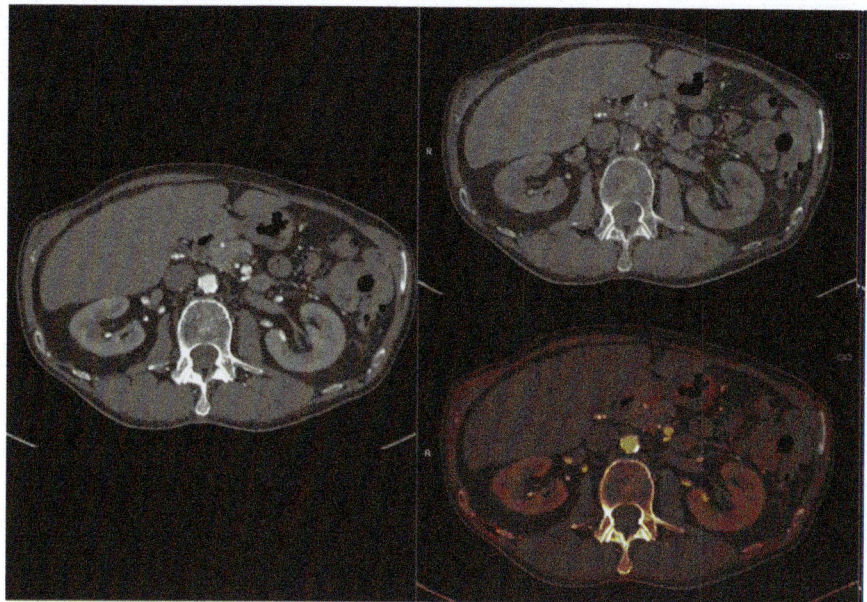

Fig. 1.8 Clinical example acquired with the Twin Beam DE technique: Mixed image corresponding to a standard 120 kV image (*left*), virtual noncontrast image (*top right*), and iodine overlay map (*bottom right*) (Courtesy of Erlangen University, Germany)

This technology provides DE data in the full SFOV of 50 cm diameter, and the radiation dose to the patient can be optimized by means of anatomical tube current modulation. The temporal registration of both data sets is good and allows acquisitions with contrast agent even in the arterial phase. As a downside, the spectral separation is worse than with approaches using two different kV settings of the x-ray tube. Furthermore, a powerful x-ray tube is required because the pre-filtration absorbs a considerable portion of the x-ray flux, and the maximum volume coverage speed is limited. Fig. 1.8 shows a clinical example acquired with the Twin Beam technique.

1.5.4 Dual Source CT

Another technical solution developed in the last years in order to acquire DECT scan data is the Dual Source CT (DSCT) [1–5]. The principle is simple: Two different x-ray spectra can be obtained by using two independent x-ray tubes, each one with its proper x-ray tube voltage ΔV and tube current values [1–5]. The x-rays tubes of DSCT scanners, together with their corresponding detectors, are mounted onto the same gantry with an angular offset of about 90°, and both measurement systems acquire scan data simultaneously at the same anatomical level [1–5] (Fig. 1.9).

The first generation of DSCT scanners was introduced into clinical practice in 2006 (*Somatom Definition, Siemens Healthcare, Forchheim, Germany,* with 2×64

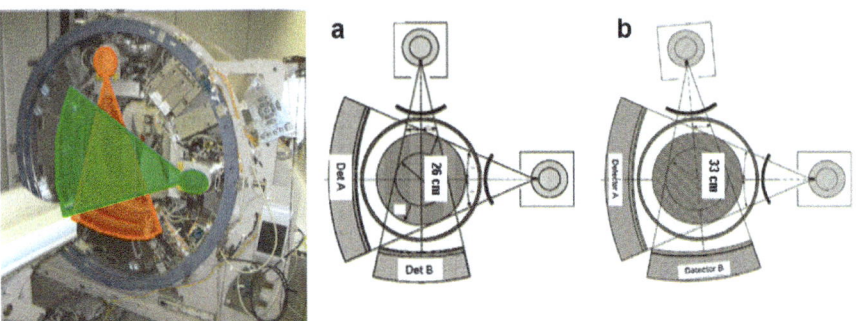

Fig. 1.9 Principle of dual source CT. (**a**) First generation. (**b**) Second generation. The third generation has a further enlarged SFOV of detector B (35.6 cm)

slices and 0.33 s gantry rotation time), the second generation in 2009 (*Somatom Definition Flash, Siemens Healthcare, Forchheim, Germany,* with 2 × 128 slices and 0.28 s gantry rotation time), and the third generation in 2014 (*Somatom Definition Force, Siemens Healthcare, Forchheim, German,* with 2 × 192 slices and 0.25 s gantry rotation time).

With the two x-ray tubes of a DSCT, two different x-ray spectra can be generated simultaneously with independent values of tube current (e.g., 80 and 140 kV) and tube voltage. It is therefore easily possible to balance the radiation dose of the low kV and the high kV data, to optimize the radiation dose to the patient by means of anatomical tube current modulation (*CARE Dose4D; Siemens Medical Solution, Forchheim, Germany*) [4] and to obtain two independent image data sets [2, 3, 5].

As another advantage, the spectral separation can be improved by introducing a dedicated tin pre-filter into the tube collimator housing of the high kV beam when needed. The quality of DECT examinations relies on the effective separation of the energy spectra. More spectral overlap and worse energy separation mean less efficient and less precise tissue differentiation, which has to be compensated by increased radiation dose. The second-generation DSCT uses an additional tin filter (Sn) with a thickness of 0.4 mm to shift the mean energy of the 140 kV spectrum from 69 to 89 keV, see Fig. 1.10. The mean energy of the 80 kV spectrum is 52 keV.

The tin filter has several benefits. It increases the spectral separation between the low- and the high-energy spectrum, it narrows the 140 kV spectrum (which results in better dose efficiency and less beam hardening artifacts) and it reduces cross-scattering. The third-generation DSCT SOMATOM Force further improves spectral separation by providing 150 kV x-ray tube voltage with more aggressive tin pre-filtration (0.6 mm) to acquire the high-energy CT data. 70, 80 and 90 kV x-ray tube voltage are available to acquire the low-energy CT data, with sufficient power reserves to scan adults and larger patients [9]. The final result is an improved tissue contrast between two materials in the CT images [2, 3]. It has been demonstrated that the DE iodine ratio, i.e., the CT number of iodine at low kV divided by the CT number at high kV is a good indicator for spectral separation and the quality of a DE CT scan [9]. The DE ratio increases from about 1.9 to 2 at the standard 80 kV/140 kV

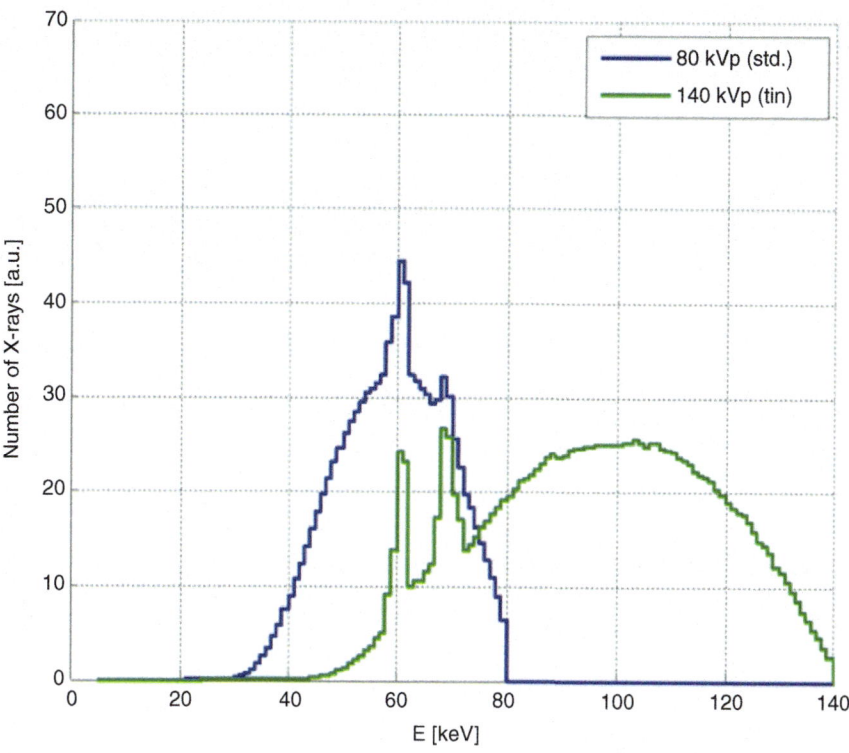

Fig. 1.10 Standard 80 kV spectrum and 140 kV spectrum with 0.4 mm tin pre-filtration (normalized to equal intensity). The tin pre-filtration absorbs x-ray quanta with energies below 50 keV. It shifts the mean energy of the 140 kV spectrum to 89 keV to improve the spectral separation in DE scans (compare to Fig. 1.2)

x-ray tube voltage combination to about 3.4 if 80 kV is combined with 150 kV and 0.6 mm tin pre-filtration. Spectral pre-filtration of the high kV beam is beneficial for DE CT at low radiation dose. Several authors have meanwhile demonstrated dual source DE CT scanning with no dose penalty compared with standard single energy CT [10, 11]. A comprehensive overview on radiation dose in DE CT is given in [12].

Image noise and radiation dose in dual source DE CT can be further reduced by iterative reconstruction methods (*SAFIRE or ADMIRE; Siemens Healthcare, Forchheim, Germany*) [3]. To reduce the image noise in particular in the low kV images, a CT detector with significantly reduced electronics noise was introduced (*Stellar Detector; Siemens Healthcare, Forchheim, Germany*). This detector minimizes electronics noise and cross-talk by direct integration of Si photodiodes and analog-digital converters in the same Si substrate [3, 7].

As a downside, scan data in dual source DE imaging are acquired with a 90° offset of both measurement systems. Unlike with other approaches, such as rapid kV switching, high-energy projections and the corresponding low-energy projections are not simultaneously measured at the same projection angle, and raw data-based DE

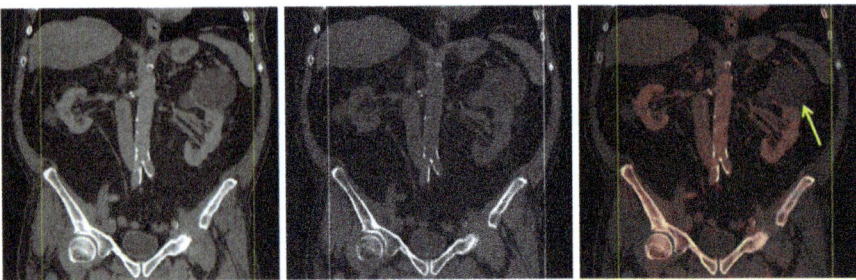

Fig. 1.11 DE CT scan acquired with a third-generation DSCT scanner at 90 kV/Sn 150 kV. $\text{CTDI}_{vol} = 12.85$ mGy. *Left*: mixed image. *Center*: virtual noncontrast image. *Right*: iodine overlay map. A large kidney cyst is characterized by a lack of iodine enhancement (*arrow*) (Courtesy of University of Mannheim, Germany)

algorithms are difficult to realize. DE algorithms are therefore image-based. Furthermore, images of moving objects may show different motion artifacts, which can result in registration problems and affect the material decomposition of the DE images. In practice, however, this problem is mitigated by the good temporal resolution of DSCT and by nonrigid registration of low kV and high kV images [3, 4]. Another disadvantage is the smaller SFOV of the second measurement system in a DSCT scanner. While the first measurement system covers the full SFOV of 50 cm diameter, the diameter of the second measurement system is limited to 26 cm (first-generation DSCT), 33 cm (second-generation DSCT) or 35.6 cm (third-generation DSCT) because of space limitations on the gantry ring. While images can be reconstructed in the full 50 cm SFOV, DE information is only available in the smaller SFOV. This can be problematic for bigger and obese patients [2, 3, 5]. A third challenge is cross-scattered radiation, i.e., scattered radiation originating from x-ray tube A and detected by detector B and vice versa. Cross-scattered radiation may cause cupping and streaking artifacts, and it can reduce image contrasts. In DSCT systems, it is corrected for by means of measurement-based or model-based correction algorithms.

Fig. 1.11 shows a clinical example of a DE CT scan acquired with a third-generation DSCT system.

1.5.5 CT Systems with Dual Layer Detector

Single source CT systems with dual layer detector technology were commercially introduced in 2013 (*IQon; Philips Healthcare, Eindhoven, The Netherlands*). A dual layer detector consists of two conventional scintillation detectors, one placed on top of the other. The x-ray tube is operated at a tube voltage of 120 or 140 kV. The top layer of the detector predominantly absorbs lower energy x-ray photons, while the bottom layer detects the remaining higher energy x-ray photons. Therefore, the signals of the two detector layers correspond to different effective x-ray spectra with different mean energies [2–5, 7]. To improve energy separation, both detector layers can consist of different scintillation materials.

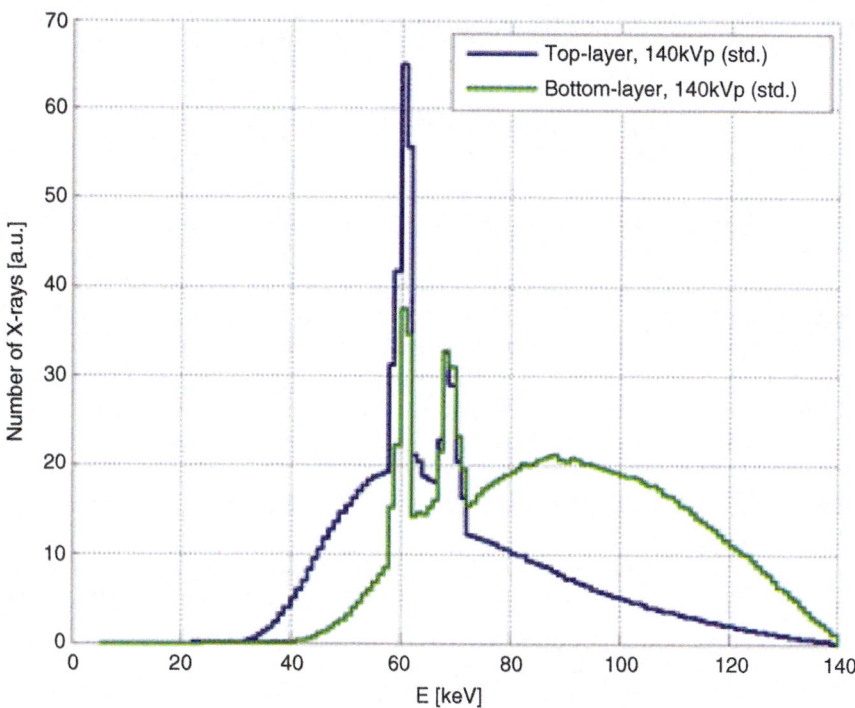

Fig. 1.12 Low-energy and high-energy spectra registered by a dual layer detector with a 1 mm thick ZnSe top layer and a GOS bottom layer, as an example for the spectral separation achievable with the dual layer approach. A primary 140 kV x-ray spectrum was used

Dual layer detectors enable acquisition of DE data with standard CT systems within full SFOV. Radiation dose can be adapted to the planned examination and the patient's body habitus by using anatomical x-ray tube current modulation. DE data can be acquired at short gantry rotation times which are a prerequisite for the examination of moving organs such as the heart. Raw data-based evaluation methods are feasible, and there are no registration problems or problems with motion artifacts because of the simultaneous acquisition of low-energy and high-energy data.

As a downside, the spectral separation is inferior to dual energy approaches relying on two different kV settings (e.g., 80 and 140 kV). With different kV settings, there is no spectral overlap in the keV range between low and high tube voltage (between 80 and 140 keV in case of 80 and 140 kV tube voltage). The top layer of a dual layer detector primarily absorbs low-energy x-ray quanta; it does, however, also absorb higher energy photons. Therefore, low-energy and high-energy spectra overlap in the entire spectral range, see Fig. 1.12.

Furthermore, it is not easily possible to apply strategies such as low kV imaging (at 70 or 80 kV) to reduce radiation dose in pediatric CT or in CT angiographic examinations, because the quantum efficiency of a dual layer detector is optimized for 120 or 140 kV.

1.6   Applications of Dual Energy CT

The processing of DE data to generate material selective or pseudo-monoenergetic images, can either be performed in the raw data space or in the image data space. Then, low-energy and high-energy images are reconstructed as a first step, and the DE processing is applied to these images. Raw data–based evaluation is often considered superior to image data–based evaluation, because image-based methods are claimed to be limited by beam hardening problems. However, under conditions that are typically fulfilled in modern CT systems image-based methods are practically equivalent.

One prerequisite for image-based material decomposition is the validity of the so-called thin absorber model. If we use water and iodine as the base materials for image-based DE evaluation, the maximum iodine attenuation is expected to be so small that it is valid to assume a linear contribution to the total attenuation. The thin absorber model holds for iodine samples up to 5000 HU cm in water, which corresponds to the clinical situation of an object with 200 HU iodine enhancement and 25 cm diameter.

In addition, neither the CT value of water nor the CT value of a small iodine sample shall depend on the position within the scanned object. This is typically achieved if the scanner is equipped with an appropriate bowtie filter and if the patient is centered within the SFOV.

In practice, electronics noise, scanner calibration, stability of emitted spectra, cone beam effects, and scattered radiation can have a larger impact on the obtained results than the analysis method.

In the following, we mainly describe image-based techniques for DE processing and focus on applications relevant for oncological imaging.

1.6.1   Pseudo Mono-energetic Images

To obtain pseudo mono-energetic images at arbitrary energies from the polychromatic low-energy and high-energy images, we assume the object to consist of only two materials in variable concentrations. Typically, water and iodine are used as base materials. The concentrations of both materials in each image pixel are calculated by a two-material decomposition, multiplied with predicted CT numbers per concentration at the desired x-ray energy, and summed up to the final mono-energetic image. Other materials will contribute to both base material images, their CT numbers may therefore not reflect the actual enhancement of the respective material at the desired energy.

In a simple application, pseudo mono-energetic images are computed in an energy range (e.g, from 40 to 150 keV in steps of 1 keV), and the CT number of a region of interest is displayed as a function of the keV. This leads to material specific curves on a Cartesian graph, see Fig. 1.13.

Object regions composed of materials with high atomic number, such as calcium and tissues containing iodinated contrast agent, will show a significant increase of

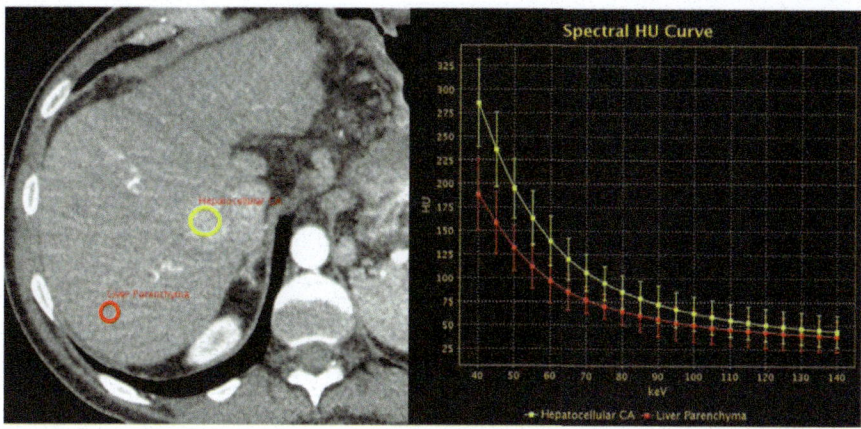

Fig. 1.13 Image obtained from a DE acquisition using rapid kV-switching in a patient with hepatocellular carcinoma (*left*). The CT numbers in two regions of interest (normal tissue, *red circle* and hepatocellular carcinoma, *yellow circle*) are displayed as a function of the energy keV of pseudo mono-energetic images (*right*). Regions containing iodinated contrast agent show a significant increase of the CT number with decreasing keV (From [14])

the CT number at lower keV. Object regions containing materials with low atomic number, on the other hand, will show only small variations of the CT number as a function of the keV. The CT number of fat will decrease with decreasing keV. In several clinical studies, the investigators have meanwhile tried to characterize lesions by their specific curves in the CT-number versus keV diagram [13].

Pseudo mono-energetic images may be used in oncological studies to benefit from the increased iodine contrast at lower keV, to increase the conspicuity of certain lesions. Unfortunately, using traditional two-material decomposition techniques, the image noise increases significantly for energies far away from the mean energy of the respective polychromatic input images (about 60–70 keV). Recently an algorithm (Mono+, Siemens Healthcare, Forchheim, Germany) was introduced that reduces image noise in pseudo mono-energetic images at low and high keV [15]. Using this approach, the lower spatial frequencies of images at the target keV and the higher spatial frequencies of images at optimal keV from a noise perspective are combined. As a result, the object information (which is contained in the lower spatial frequencies) at the target keV is combined with low image noise.

It has been shown [15] that it may be more efficient to perform DE scans and compute pseudo mono-energetic images at 40 keV using Mono + to optimize iodine CNR than to perform scans at 80 or 100 kV, which has been the established and recommended method to improve iodine CNR to date. Figure 1.14 shows a clinical example for the application of mono-energetic imaging at low keV.

Mono-energetic images at the other end of the keV-spectrum, at very high keV, may be used to efficiently reduce metal artifacts, as long as they are caused by beam hardening and not by photon starvation. This has been demonstrated for hip replacements [16] and posterior spinal fusion implants [17].

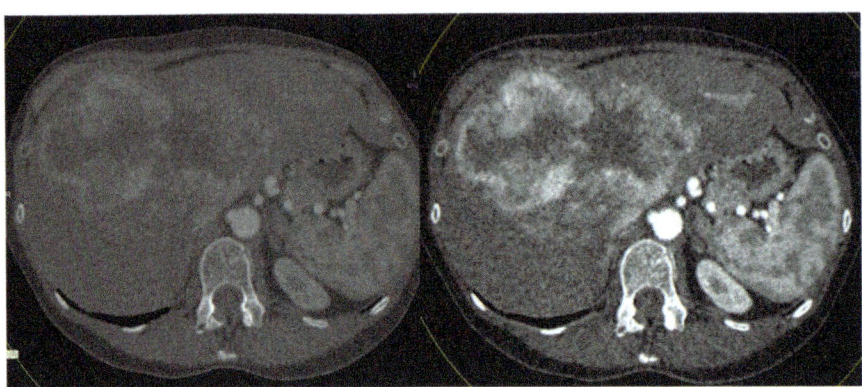

Fig. 1.14 DE image acquired on a third-generation DSCT scanner at 100 kV/Sn 150 kV. *Left*: Mixed image, corresponding to a standard 120 kV acquisition. *Right*: Pseudo mono-energetic image using the Mono+technique at 40 keV. Note the significantly increased iodine CNR (Courtesy of University Hospital Zurich, Switzerland)

1.6.2 Virtual Nonenhanced Images and Iodine Maps

Using the polychromatic low kV and high kV images, iodine can be subtracted from a contrast-enhanced CT scan. As a result, both virtual nonenhanced CT images and iodine maps quantifying and visualizing the iodine content per image pixel are obtained. The underlying technique is a modified three-material decomposition, see the diagram in Fig. 1.15 which shows the CT number of each image pixel at low kV as a function of its CT number at high kV. If the three-material decomposition is applied to liver imaging, fat, soft tissue and iodine are used as base materials. Image pixels containing mixtures of fat and soft tissue are located along a line between pure fat and pure soft tissue. If iodinated contrast agent is added, the respective data points in the CT-number diagram move in the direction of the iodine enhancement vector. To extract the iodine, each pixel in the CT-number diagram is projected onto the line between fat and soft tissue along the direction of the iodine enhancement vector. The length of the displacement vector represents the enhancement attributed to iodine in that pixel (see the example in Fig. 1.15).

The iodine enhancement values for all pixels ("iodine content") are displayed in the iodine map. It can be subtracted from the contrast-enhanced image to provide a virtual nonenhanced image. The iodine map can provide quantitative information about the iodine content in mg/ml. If the three-material decomposition is applied to other abdominal imaging tasks, e.g., kidney imaging where characterization of cysts may play a role, water, soft tissue, and iodine are used as base materials. This way, a water value of 0 HU in the virtual nonenhanced image is ensured.

Virtual noncontrast images calculated from DE scans may in some cases replace true noncontrast CT images. Avoiding additional CT scans without contrast agent may reduce the radiation dose to the patient. The use of virtual noncontrast images in oncology has been described for the differentiation of liver and kidney tumors

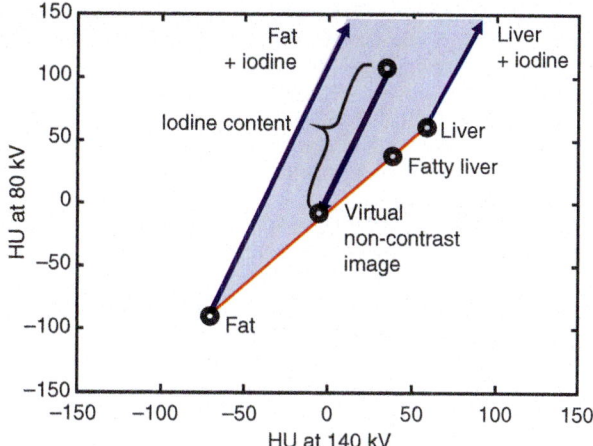

Fig. 1.15 Principle of image-based three-material decomposition for a dual energy liver scan to obtain a virtual noncontrast image and an iodine map

and adrenal masses. Iodine maps have been used to characterize the local blood supply of tumors with the goal of an earlier assessment of the response to anti-angiogenesis therapies (for an overview, refer to [5, 6, 18–21]).

A variant of the three-material decomposition method with air, soft tissue, and iodine as base materials has been used to compute iodine maps of the lung parenchyma as a surrogate parameter for the local blood volume. Most commonly, this technique is used to visualize the extent of perfusion defects caused by pulmonary embolism. DE CT of the lung, however, has also other applications. It has been shown to improve the diagnosis of acute and chronic PEs, other vascular disorders, lung malignancies, and parenchymal diseases [22, 23].

To summarize, DE CT is an innovative technology, readily available in clinical practice, which may significantly affect the management of oncologic patients.

Literature

1. Saba L, Suri J (2014) Multi-detector CT imaging: abdomen, pelvis and CAD applications. In: Flohr T, Schmidt B (eds) Dual energy computed tomography: tissue characterization. Taylor & Francis Group, LLC, Boca Raton, Fl, pp 553–562
2. Johnson TRC (2012) Dual-energy CT: general principles. AJR Am J Roentgenol 199:S3–S8
3. Marin D et al (2014) State of the art: dual-energy CT of the abdomen. Radiology 271(2)
4. Aran S et al (2014) Dual-energy computed tomography (DECT) in emergency radiology: basic principles, techniques, and limitations. Emerg Radiol 21:391–405
5. Agrawal MD et al (2014) Oncologic applications of dual-energy CT in the abdomen. Radiographics 34:589–612
6. Simons D et al (2014) Recent developments of dual-energy CT in oncology. Eur Radiol 24:930–939
7. Kraśnicki T et al (2012) Novel clinical applications of dual energy computed tomography. Adv Clin Exp Med 21(6):831–841
8. Kaza RK, Platt JF, Cohan RH, Caoili EM, Al-Hawary MM, Wasnik A (2012) Dual-energy CT with single- and dual-source scanners: current applications in evaluating the genitourinary tract. Radiographics 32(2):353–369

9. Krauss B, Grant KL, Schmidt BT, Flohr TG (2015) The importance of spectral separation: an assessment of dual-energy spectral separation for quantitative ability and dose efficiency. Invest Radiol 50(2):114–118

10. Schenzle JC, Sommer WH, Neumaier K et al (2010) Dual energy CT of the chest: how about the dose? Invest Radiol 45:347–353

11. Bauer RW, Kramer S, Renker M et al (2011) Dose and image quality at CT pulmonary angiography: comparison of first and second generation dual energy CT and 64-slice CT. Eur Radiol 21:2139–2147

12. Henzler T, Fink C, Schoenberg SO, Schoepf UJ (2012) Dual energy CT: radiation dose aspects. AJR Am J Roentgenol 199:S16–S25

13. Liu X, Ouyang D, Li H, Zhang R, Lv Y, Yang A, Xie C (2015) Papillary thyroid cancer: dual-energy spectral CT quantitative parameters for preoperative diagnosis of metastasis to the cervical lymph nodes. Radiology 275(1):167–176

14. Morgan MD (2010) GE Healthcare case study GSI lesion characterization

15. Grant KL, Flohr TG, Krauss B, Sedlmair M, Thomas C, Schmidt B (2014) Assessment of an advanced image-based technique to calculate virtual monoenergetic computed tomographic images from a dual-energy examination to improve contrast-to-noise ratio in examinations using iodinated contrast media. Invest Radiol 49(9):586–592

16. Lewis M, Reid K, Toms AP (2013) Reducing the effects of metal artefact using high keV monoenergetic reconstruction of dual energy CT (DECT) in hip replacements. Skeletal Radiol 42(2):275–282

17. Guggenberger R, Winklhofer S, Osterhoff G, Wanner GA, Fortunati M, Andreisek G, Alkadhi H, Stolzmann P (2012) Metallic artefact reduction with monoenergetic dual-energy CT: systematic ex vivo evaluation of posterior spinal fusion implants from various vendors and different spine levels. Eur Radiol 22(11):2357–2364

18. De Cecco CN, Darnell A, Rengo M, Muscogiuri G, Bellini D, Ayuso C, Laghi A (2012) Dual-energy CT: oncologic applications. AJR Am J Roentgenol 199(5 Suppl):S98–S105

19. Uhrig M, Sedlmair M, Schlemmer HP, Hassel JC, Ganten M (2013) Monitoring targeted therapy using dual-energy CT: semi-automatic RECIST plus supplementary functional information by quantifying iodine uptake of melanoma metastases. Cancer Imaging 13(3):306–313

20. Knobloch G, Jost G, Huppertz A, Hamm B, Pietsch H (2014) Dual-energy computed tomography for the assessment of early treatment effects of regorafenib in a preclinical tumor model: comparison with dynamic contrast-enhanced CT and conventional contrast-enhanced single-energy CT. Eur Radiol 24(8):1896–1905

21. Apfaltrer P, Meyer M, Meier C, Henzler T, Barraza JM Jr, Dinter DJ, Hohenberger P, Schoepf UJ, Schoenberg SO, Fink C (2012) Contrast-enhanced dual-energy CT of gastrointestinal stromal tumors: is iodine-related attenuation a potential indicator of tumor response? Invest Radiol 47(1):65–70

22. Lu GM, Zhao Y, Zhang LJ, Schoepf UJ (2012) Dual-energy CT of the lung. AJR Am J Roentgenol 199(5 Suppl):S40–S53

23. Zhang LJ, Yang GF, Wu SY, Xu J, Lu GM, Schoepf UJ (2013) Dual-energy CT imaging of thoracic malignancies. Cancer Imaging 13:81–91

Dual Energy CT Postprocessing and Images Analysis Strategies in Oncologic Imaging

2

Hua-Dan Xue and Liang Zhu

2.1 Introduction

Multiple detector CT (MDCT) has been the first-choice imaging modality for many oncologic applications, including lesion detection, classification, radiological staging, follow-up, and treatment effect monitoring. However, in some special clinical settings, MDCT remains problematic, or inconclusive. A classic example is high-density cystic-appearing renal lesions. Could it be a hemorrhagic or high protein-content cyst, or an enhancing tumor? Another problem we have, for instance, is Lipiodol treated hepatic cell carcinoma. The high-density iodine-containing Lipiodol masked the enhancing portion of the residual lesion, making it extremely difficult to evaluate treatment effect. DECT material decomposition capability would be a potential solution for these clinical dilemmas.

With single-energy CT, differentiation and quantification of different tissue types is difficult, since CT number measured in a voxel is not specific for any given material, but a function of the material composition, the photon energy used for scanning and the density of each material. In dual-energy CT, images are acquired with two distinguished photon energies. This unique feature enables several sets of postprocessed images, which provide additional information with clinical significance. With DECT, the exact content of each voxel could be calculated, assuming that it is composed of 2 or 3 known materials. A linear-attenuation coefficient map of each voxel could also be generated, with which virtual monochromatic spectral images (VMS) could be created in a wide range of photon energies.

H.-D. Xue (✉) • L. Zhu
Department of Radiology, Peking Medical College Hospital,
Shuaifuyuan No1, Dongcheng District, Peking 100730, China
e-mail: Bjdanna95@hotmail.com; Zhuliang_pumc@163.com

© Springer International Publishing Switzerland 2015
C.N. De Cecco et al. (eds.), *Dual Energy CT in Oncology*,
DOI 10.1007/978-3-319-19563-6_2

21

2.2   Additional Information from Dual-Energy Image Acquisition

2.2.1   Linear and Nonlinear Blended Images

With dual-energy CT scanning, both high-energy and low-energy images are acquired, which could directly be used for radiologic diagnosis. However, low-energy images (i.e. 80 kVp) have higher "graininess" and a more compromised overall image quality, although iodine contrast is more prominent. High-energy images are smoother and of less noise; however, the contrast between different tissues is reduced, making some lesions less conspicuous. To achieve a better balance between image quality and lesion contrast, images could be blended utilizing information from both low energy and high energy (Figs. 2.1 and 2.2). The "mixed" images could be used for routine clinical diagnosis [5, 24].

Linear blending is simply combining the high- and low-energy imaging set with a given linear ratio (e.g. $\lambda = 0.3$ means 30 % image information was derived from the low-energy data set whereas the rest 70 % was from the high-energy set). It could be done within minutes on the console [10]. The blending ratio could be set up according to the preference of radiologists in practice but usually is not changed on a case-by-case basis [24].

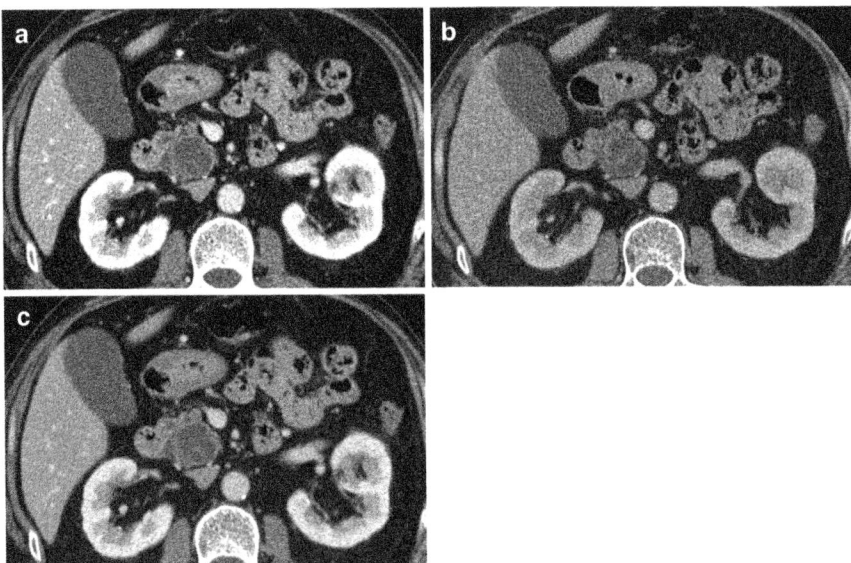

Fig. 2.1 80 kVp (**a**), Sn140 kVp (**b**) and weighted average (WA) 120 kVp (**c**) portal venous phase images of the upper abdomen, demonstrating a low attenuation cystic mass in the uncinate process of the pancreas. Surgical pathology proved intraductal papillary mucinous neoplasm (IPMN). Note that liver parenchyma and liver cortex appear much brighter and sharper on low-energy images. Weighted average images achieved a better balance between contrast and image "softness"

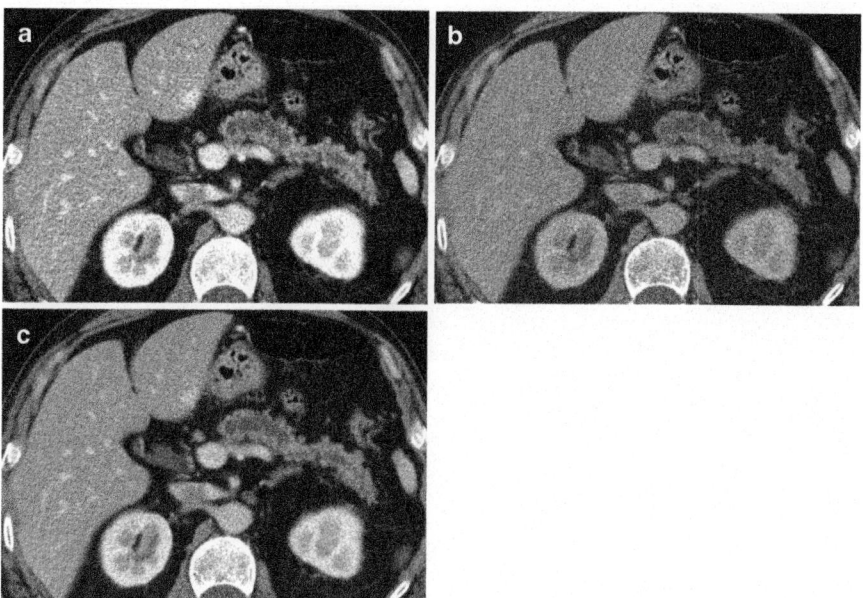

Fig. 2.2 Same case of Fig. 2.1. The dilated main pancreatic duct surrounded by atrophic pancreatic parenchyma is better displayed on the weighted average (WA) 120 kVp (**c**) compared with the 80 kVp (**a**) and Sn140 Vp (**b**) data sets

Another more sophisticated method is to blend the two image sets in a nonlinear fashion. A comparison of several different nonlinear image blending algorithms has shown that moidal blending provides the optimal image characteristics [9]. This approach adopts low-energy data for those areas that show more iodine enhancement, and utilize high-energy data for those image regions that show less or no iodine enhancement. Nonlinear blending is based on a more complicated algorithm and is available only on dedicate postprocessing workstations.

2.2.2   Material Decomposition

Different algorithms were adopted by different vendors for material decomposition with dual-energy CT. With dual-source dual-energy CT (Siemens), a three-material decomposition (default set: iodine, soft tissue, and fat) algorithm was applied, processing data in the image space. The numerical stability of three-material decomposition is partly based on dual-energy ratio of the material composition [11]. For materials with similar dual-energy ratios, this algorithm becomes much less stable [14]. However, it has been proved to work well only when one of the assumed three materials has a very different dual-energy ratio compared to others, such as iodine. To decrease the photon energy overlap at two tube potentials could also increase the stability of material decomposition capability. The second generation dual-source

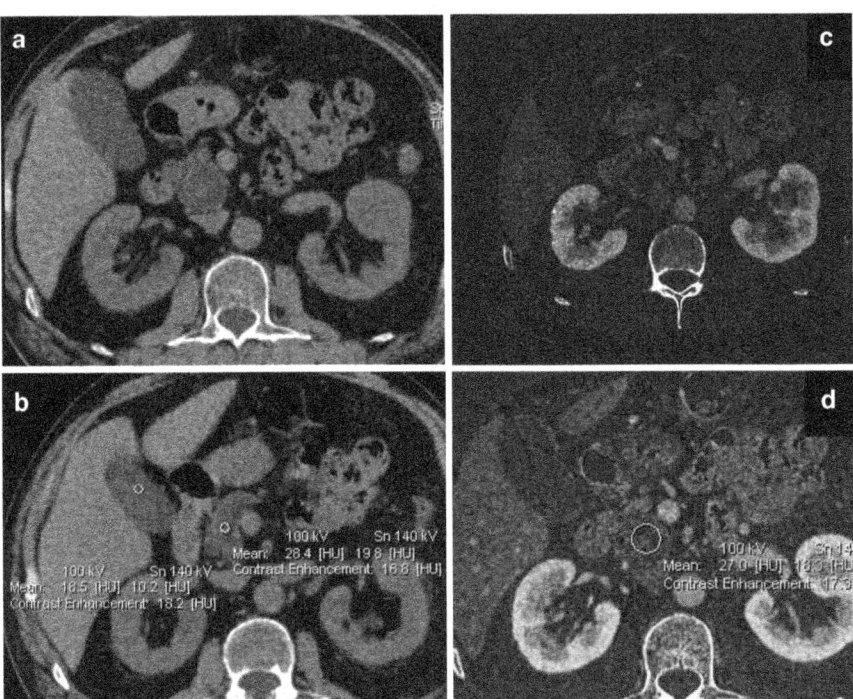

Fig. 2.3 Liver VNC postprocessing software displays virtual noncontrast (VNC) and iodine map side by side. VNC may replace real noncontrast acquisition (**a**), and attenuation values can be directly measured (**b**). Iodine map can be used to directly visualize iodine content in the lesion (**c**), and measure it with a ROI (**d**). In the iodine map, the details of the lesion can be appreciated more clearly. The low attenuation content within the lesion is iodine free, but the enhancing septa clearly contain iodine on the map (**e**), well depicting a complex cystic mass with multiple thin septa

dual-energy CT (Siemens Definition Flash) has accomplished this by adding an extra tin filter to the high energy tube [26].

Single-source fast-kilovoltage switching DECT (GE) adopted a two-material decomposition algorithm in the projection domain. It assumes that the scanned object is composed of two base materials (water and iodine as the default pair). Images acquired at high- and low-energy is postprocessed to generate iodine-based and water-based images, similar to virtual noncontrast (VNC) images and iodine map in its dual-source DECT counterpart (Fig. 2.3). Theoretically, projection-domain decomposition has its unique advantage in that beam-hardening effects could be avoided. However, motion artifact, which may destroy the data consistency between the low- and high-energy data, could degrade image quality with this algorithm.

2.2.3   Virtual Monochromatic Images

With dual-energy acquisition, the material composition of each voxel of the scanned object could be calculated. With two (or three) known material bases each in a specific fraction, a linear-attenuation coefficient map of each voxel could be generated,

Table 2.1 Commercially available DECT software used in clinical oncologic radiology

Image types	Dual-source dual-energy CT	Single-source dual-energy CT
Image blending		
Linear blending	(console automatic reconstruction) Weighted average (WA) images	–
Nonlinear blending	Syngo Optimum contrast	–
Material decomposition		
Pair of virtual noncontrast (VNC) image and iodine map	Syngo Liver VNC (default or modified), with or without 3D volumetric application	Iodine-based and water-based images
VNC, iodine overlay together with bone removal	Syngo dual-energy brain hemorrhage	–
Virtual monochromatic images		
40–140 keV energy-selective image series	Syngo DE-CT monoenergetic	Virtual monochromatic (VMC) images

at any energy within the diagnostic energy range. Therefore, a dual-energy data set could be postprocessed into a range of virtual monochromatic (VMC) images, with an automatically generated spectral attenuation curve, allowing for selection of the "optimum contrast" or "lowest noise" set for clinical diagnosis.

The most commonly used DECT postprocessing software in oncologic image, which are currently commercially available are summarized in Table. 2.1.

2.3   Objective Evaluation of Postprocessed Images

2.3.1   Image Noise, SNR, and CNR

One of the major concerns with DECT images is the image noise and lesion-to-background contrast, compared to images acquired with single-energy CT (SECT) at comparable radiation dose.

Image noise, which could be subjectively perceived by radiologists as the image "graininess," could also be objectively measured and compared in parallel in images acquired with different scanning procedures. Generally it is defined as the standard deviation of attenuation in the retroperitoneal fat or subcutaneous fat in the abdominal wall, measured with a standardized region of interest (ROI) of 1 cm² area [6, 8, 23]. Sometimes it is also measured in the muscle [20] or air adjacent to the scanned object [30].

Signal-to-noise ratio (SNR) could also be evaluated in each organ of interest. With a standardized ROI, SNR is calculated by dividing the mean attenuation number by the corresponding standard deviation [1, 32].

Contrast-to-noise ratio (CNR) is a quantitative parameter with even greater clinical significance. Images with higher CNR are always desired since lesions are more readily detectable when they appear in higher contrast with the background normal tissue. CNR in the same object scanned with DECT and SECT has been investigated in several phantom studies [15] as well as in many clinical oncologic researches [16, 20, 28, 30, 31]. First, ROIs are selected in an area representing the lesion, as well as an area representing the "background," be it liver parenchyma, pancreatic parenchyma, or renal parenchyma adjacent to but independent from the lesion. Then CNR is calculated as follows:

$$CNR = \left(ROI_{lesion} - ROI_{background} \right) / \sigma ROI_{background}$$

ROI_{lesion} is the attenuation value of the lesion, $ROI_{background}$ is the attenuation value of the background and σ is the standard deviation.

Such quantitative image evaluations have been widely carried out in various organs and disease conditions. Zhang et al. compared SNR and CNR of liver lesions on TNC and VNC acquired in both arterial phase and portal venous phase, in 102 patients with suspected liver disease. They reported that SNR was significantly higher on VNC, and the highest CNR was achieved with VNCa [32]. Kim et al. compared CNR in fused image data using linear blending method and nonlinear blending method with different weighted factors in a renal phantom and found nonlinear blended image sets the most preferred one [15]. Similar image analysis strategy was adopted with evaluation of hypovascular liver metastasis [28], renal masses [8], laryngeal and hypopharyngeal cancer [19] and lung cancer [17].

2.3.2   Lesion Enhancement and Iodine Concentration

Radiological diagnosis or lesion classification is largely based on lesion enhancement. The behavior of a specific lesion after contrast administration is critical for differential diagnosis. Take renal lesions for example, almost all enhancing lesions are potentially neoplastic. Lesion enhancement could be measured with SECT; however, problems exist in some clinical cases. For SECT, ROIs are placed manually on nonenhanced images as well as enhanced images, and potential misregistration could lead to a false judgment [4].

With dual-energy acquisition, images could be obtained with iodine content of each voxel extracted and independently displayed (iodine map). By placing a ROI on the postprocessed VNC/iodine map images, the iodine distribution within the lesion could be readily documented.

Validation studies of iodine quantification within lesions have been carried out in phantom studies [4, 21] as well as clinical cases [17, 22], and its ability to enhance diagnostic accuracy and confidence has also been evaluated [2, 8, 16].

2.3.3   Spectral HU Curve and Z_{eff}

On fast-kilovoltage switching single-source dual-energy CT, a real-time interactive display of virtual monochromatic (VMC) images could be readily displayed on an advanced workstation. The readers can place an ROI in the lesion (or the chosen "background"), and a spectral HU curve will be automatically generated, by plotting the mean CT value within the ROI under discrete monochromatic energies (usually from 40 to 140 keV), and the effective atomic number (Z_{eff}) within the ROI is simultaneously displayed. Z_{eff} and the characteristics of spectral HU curve may help to distinguish different lesions and has been investigated in many clinical settings, including renal stone composition determination [18, 27], classification of benign and malignant thyroid nodules [22], differentiation between benign and malignant pathologies for patients with palpable masses in the neck [29] and so on. In those published work, the curve characteristics under investigation included the difference between the highest and lowest attenuation value, asymptote, decay and the difference in ranges between lesion and tissue background. And it has been shown that the difference in ranges between lesion and paraspinal muscle might facilitate clinical diagnosis in neck masses [29], and the HU curve slope (λHU) and Z_{eff} are significantly different in benign and malignant thyroid nodules. However, researches concerning the value of spectral curve and effective atomic numbers remain limited in oncologic applications.

2.4   Subjective Analysis of Postprocessed Images

2.4.1   Overall Image Quality and Noise

The subjective image quality and noise is often compared between DECT postprocessed images and conventional SECT images, usually with a scoring system. The image quality is rated with a 3–5 point scales, from "not interpretable" to "excellent" [7, 8], while image noise could be rated from "inferior compared to conventional images" to "superior to conventional images" [3]. For dual-source dual-energy CT, especially the first-generation scanner, tube B has a limited field of view (26 cm). This becomes problematic for thoracic and abdominal scans, especially for larger sized patients. By placing the target organ in the centre of scanning field could partially fix this problem (i.e. for patients suspected of liver disease); however, for patients with renal lesions, the contralateral kidney might be excluded. Another problem is that fused image or material decomposition images will be incomplete, since the excluded part only has information from the single energy (higher energy) portion. The second-generation dual-source DECT has a larger FOV, but incomplete image fusion still exists in patients with greater body mass index (BMI). Therefore, the exclusion of important abdominal organs is also an aspect of investigation [6]. Single-source DECT doesn't have such FOV limits. It should also be noticed that for dual-source DECT, when readers were asked to compare image quality and noise between SECT and DECT images, it is often difficult to mask the origin of images to them, since the incomplete margin of fused images is easy to tell.

2.4.2 Lesion Conspicuity

In the evaluation of the potential of virtual noncontrast images (VNC) to replace true noncontrast images (TNC), or in the selection of optimized images for clinical interpretation among a range of postprocessed images, lesion conspicuity is one of the major considerations. It is usually determined by 2 or more radiologists, who read those images independently or in consensus, and give out a score for each of them [15, 20, 28]. With an improved delineation of tumor margins, tumor invasion depth, or the adjacent organs involvement could be more confidently determined. Lesion contour delineation could be rated with scales [30]. The presence or absence of transmural tumor invasion or adjacent organ involvement could be interpreted on different image sets, including conventional SECT and postprocessed DECT images, and the diagnostic accuracy could be determined with pathologic confirmation [19, 25]. This provides direct evidence for the clinical value of DECT images.

2.4.3 Visual Lesion Enhancement

Lesion enhancement could be quantitatively determined by measurement with cursors. However, such measurement elongated case interpretation time. To determine whether postprocessed DECT could facilitate in the direct visualization of iodine-associated enhancement, a subjective analysis could provide clues. Take renal lesions for example, radiologists could review SECT images and DECT images from the same patient in a random order, and assign the lesions as "simple cysts," "hyperdense cysts," and "enhancing masses." Their diagnostic confidence could be self-evaluated and recorded. The image interpretation time could be recorded, and the diagnostic accuracy could be calculated. Several studies have reported a benefit of direct visual assistance from iodine map or iodine overlay images in differentiation between benign and malignant lesions [12, 13].

2.4.4 Detection of Calcification

For conventional SECT images, iodine and calcium could hardly be distinguished in a voxel, since they both appear hyperdense. DECT has its unique advantage for material decomposition and iodine could easily be extracted from the images. In the evaluation of ground-glass pulmonary nodules, the detection of calcification is important, since calcified nodules tend to be benign and could be safely monitored, whereas iodine-containing, enhancing nodules may need further intervention. The utility of DECT in solitary lung nodules was investigated and visual assessment of detection of calcification with VNC and TNC was performed. The number of detected calcifications was scored and the calcification size was compared between two image sets [3]. The authors found VNC allows most calcifications within a nodule to be detected.

Conclusion

Various postprocessing software for DECT are available, which provide effective tools for more accurate interpretation of clinical images. Preliminary studies have shown their additional benefits in oncologic applications. Further validation of their diagnostic value in a broader range of diseases is still needed.

References

1. Behrendt FF, Schmidt B, Plumhans C, Keil S, Woodruff SG, Ackermann D, Muhlenbruch G, Flohr T, Gunther RW, Mahnken AH (2009) Image fusion in dual energy computed tomography: effect on contrast enhancement, signal-to-noise ratio and image quality in computed tomography angiography. Invest Radiol 44:1–6
2. Brown CL, Hartman RP, Dzyubak OP, Takahashi N, Kawashima A, McCollough CH, Bruesewitz MR, Primak AM, Fletcher JG (2009) Dual-energy CT iodine overlay technique for characterization of renal masses as cyst or solid: a phantom feasibility study. Eur Radiol 19:1289–1295
3. Chae EJ, Song JW, Seo JB, Krauss B, Jang YM, Song KS (2008) Clinical utility of dual-energy CT in the evaluation of solitary pulmonary nodules: initial experience. Radiology 249:671–681
4. Chandarana H, Megibow AJ, Cohen BA, Srinivasan R, Kim D, Leidecker C, Macari M (2011) Iodine quantification with dual-energy CT: phantom study and preliminary experience with renal masses. AJR Am J Roentgenol 196:W693–W700
5. Coursey CA, Nelson RC, Boll DT, Paulson EK, Ho LM, Neville AM, Marin D, Gupta RT, Schindera ST (2010) Dual-energy multidetector CT: how does it work, what can it tell us, and when can we use it in abdominopelvic imaging? Radiographics 30:1037–1055
6. De Cecco CN et al (2010) Dual energy CT (DECT) of the liver: conventional versus virtual unenhanced images. Eur Radiol 20:2870–2875
7. Graser A et al (2010) Single-phase dual-energy CT allows for characterization of renal masses as benign or malignant. Invest Radiol 45:399–405
8. Graser A et al (2009) Dual-energy CT in patients suspected of having renal masses: can virtual nonenhanced images replace true nonenhanced images? Radiology 252:433–440
9. Holmes DR 3rd et al (2008) Evaluation of non-linear blending in dual-energy computed tomography. Eur J Radiol 68:409–413
10. Johnson TR (2012) Dual-energy CT: general principles. AJR Am J Roentgenol 199:S3–S8
11. Kachelriess M, Kalender WA (2005) Presampling, algorithm factors, and noise: considerations for CT in particular and for medical imaging in general. Med Phys 32:1321–1334
12. Kang MJ, Park CM, Lee CH, Goo JM, Lee HJ (2010) Focal iodine defects on color-coded iodine perfusion maps of dual-energy pulmonary CT angiography images: a potential diagnostic pitfall. AJR Am J Roentgenol 195:W325–W330
13. Kawai T, Shibamoto Y, Hara M, Arakawa T, Nagai K, Ohashi K (2011) Can dual-energy CT evaluate contrast enhancement of ground-glass attenuation? Phantom and preliminary clinical studies. Acad Radiol 18:682–689
14. Kelcz F, Joseph PM, Hilal SK (1979) Noise considerations in dual energy CT scanning. Med Phys 6:418–425
15. Kim KS, Lee JM, Kim SH, Kim KW, Kim SJ, Cho SH, Han JK, Choi BI (2010) Image fusion in dual energy computed tomography for detection of hypervascular liver hepatocellular carcinoma: phantom and preliminary studies. Invest Radiol 45:149–157
16. Kim SJ, Lim HK, Lee HY, Choi CG, Lee DH, Suh DC, Kim SM, Kim JK, Krauss B (2012) Dual-energy CT in the evaluation of intracerebral hemorrhage of unknown origin: differentiation between tumor bleeding and pure hemorrhage. AJNR Am J Neuroradiol 33:865–872

17. Kim YN, Lee HY, Lee KS, Seo JB, Chung MJ, Ahn MJ, Park K, Kim TS, Yi CA (2012) Dual-energy CT in patients treated with anti-angiogenic agents for non-small cell lung cancer: new method of monitoring tumor response? Korean J Radiol 13:702–710

18. Kulkarni NM, Eisner BH, Pinho DF, Joshi MC, Kambadakone AR, Sahani DV (2013) Determination of renal stone composition in phantom and patients using single-source dual-energy computed tomography. J Comput Assist Tomogr 37:37–45

19. Kuno H, Onaya H, Iwata R, Kobayashi T, Fujii S, Hayashi R, Otani K, Ojiri H, Yamanaka T, Satake M (2012) Evaluation of cartilage invasion by laryngeal and hypopharyngeal squamous cell carcinoma with dual-energy CT. Radiology 265:488–496

20. Lee SH, Lee JM, Kim KW, Klotz E, Kim SH, Lee JY, Han JK, Choi BI (2011) Dual-energy computed tomography to assess tumor response to hepatic radiofrequency ablation: potential diagnostic value of virtual noncontrast images and iodine maps. Invest Radiol 46:77–84

21. Leschka S, Stolzmann P, Baumuller S, Scheffel H, Desbiolles L, Schmid B, Marincek B, Alkadhi H (2010) Performance of dual-energy CT with tin filter technology for the discrimination of renal cysts and enhancing masses. Acad Radiol 17:526–534

22. Li M, Zheng X, Li J, Yang Y, Lu C, Xu H, Yu B, Xiao L, Zhang G, Hua Y (2012) Dual-energy computed tomography imaging of thyroid nodule specimens: comparison with pathologic findings. Invest Radiol 47:58–64

23. Lv P, Lin XZ, Chen K, Gao J (2012) Spectral CT in patients with small HCC: investigation of image quality and diagnostic accuracy. Eur Radiol 22:2117–2124

24. Megibow AJ, Sahani D (2012) Best practice: implementation and use of abdominal dual-energy CT in routine patient care. AJR Am J Roentgenol 199:S71–S77

25. Pan Z, Pang L, Ding B, Yan C, Zhang H, Du L, Wang B, Song Q, Chen K, Yan F (2013) Gastric cancer staging with dual energy spectral CT imaging. PLoS One 8:e53651

26. Primak AN, Ramirez Giraldo JC, Liu X, Yu L, McCollough CH (2009) Improved dual-energy material discrimination for dual-source CT by means of additional spectral filtration. Med Phys 36:1359–1369

27. Qu M, Ramirez-Giraldo JC, Leng S, Williams JC, Vrtiska TJ, Lieske JC, McCollough CH (2011) Dual-energy dual-source CT with additional spectral filtration can improve the differentiation of non-uric acid renal stones: an ex vivo phantom study. AJR Am J Roentgenol 196:1279–1287

28. Robinson E, Babb J, Chandarana H, Macari M (2010) Dual source dual energy MDCT: comparison of 80 kVp and weighted average 120 kVp data for conspicuity of hypo-vascular liver metastases. Invest Radiol 45:413–418

29. Srinivasan A, Parker RA, Manjunathan A, Ibrahim M, Shah GV, Mukherji SK (2013) Differentiation of benign and malignant neck pathologies: preliminary experience using spectral computed tomography. J Comput Assist Tomogr 37:666–672

30. Tawfik AM, Kerl JM, Bauer RW, Nour-Eldin NE, Naguib NN, Vogl TJ, Mack MG (2012) Dual-energy CT of head and neck cancer: average weighting of low- and high-voltage acquisitions to improve lesion delineation and image quality-initial clinical experience. Invest Radiol 47:306–311

31. Yamada Y, Jinzaki M, Tanami Y, Abe T, Kuribayashi S (2012) Virtual monochromatic spectral imaging for the evaluation of hypovascular hepatic metastases: the optimal monochromatic level with fast kilovoltage switching dual-energy computed tomography. Invest Radiol 47:292–298

32. Zhang LJ, Peng J, Wu SY, Wang ZJ, Wu XS, Zhou CS, Ji XM, Lu GM (2010) Liver virtual non-enhanced CT with dual-source, dual-energy CT: a preliminary study. Eur Radiol 20:2257–2264

Dual Energy CT in Head and Neck Tumors

3

Ahmed M. Tawfik, Boris Bodelle, and Thomas J. Vogl

3.1   Introduction

Imaging is a cornerstone in the management of head and neck cancer patients. The main role of imaging is to evaluate the true extent of disease for treatment planning. This includes accurate assessment of the size, location, and infiltration of surrounding structures. The next task of imaging is the assessment of the status of neck lymph nodes due to its importance in treatment planning and its prognostic value. In many cases, imaging may also enable a definitive diagnosis of benign processes, thus unnecessary biopsies could be avoided. In other cases, imaging may help in narrowing of the differential diagnosis, based on lesion location and other imaging features.

The complex anatomy of the head and neck region, with its several anatomic and functional subdivisions, in addition to the diversity of pathologic processes, has always been challenging for radiologists. Therefore, state-of-the-art imaging techniques should be used for head and neck imaging. Over the past decades, CT has maintained its role as the method of choice for examination of the head and neck in many institutions, mainly due to the wide availability, high experience, and short examination time. Advances in CT technology, with the introduction of multi-slice

A.M. Tawfik (✉)
Department of Diagnostic and Interventional Radiology, Faculty of Medicine,
Mansoura University, El-Gomhoreya Street, Mansoura, 35112, Egypt

Department of Diagnostic and Interventional Radiology, J.W. Goethe University of
Frankfurt, Theodor-Stern-Kai 7, Frankfurt, Germany
e-mail: Ahm_m_tawfik@hotmail.com

B. Bodelle • T.J. Vogl
Department of Diagnostic and Interventional Radiology, J.W. Goethe University of
Frankfurt, Theodor-Stern-Kai 7, Frankfurt, Germany
e-mail: bbodelle@gmail.com; T.Vogl@em.uni-frankfurt.de

© Springer International Publishing Switzerland 2015
C.N. De Cecco et al. (eds.), *Dual Energy CT in Oncology*,
DOI 10.1007/978-3-319-19563-6_3

scanners capable of isotropic imaging, have enabled increased CT resolution and multi-planar reformats. More recently, dual energy (DE) scanning became available, and new potentialities for CT imaging have emerged. Applications based on material characterization (iodine mapping), image blending and energy-specific (monochromatic imaging) applications are developing and gradually being introduced into clinical practice. The use of dual energy CT in head and neck oncology imaging aims at improving image quality, increasing lesion delineation, helping lesion characterization as well as nodal staging.

3.2   Virtual Monochromatic Images

CT exposures, including DE acquisitions, consist of photons within broad spectrum of energies (polychromatic). Using dedicated DE software, the data from the two polychromatic exposures of a DE scan could be reconstructed into a single dataset that reflects the properties of a scan with a monochromatic x-ray beam. This dataset is termed "virtual monochromatic or monoenergetic imaging." Virtual monochromatic images are generated using software based on basis material decomposition, which may be performed either in the projection (raw data) domain for single source fast-KV switching DE acquisitions or in the image domain (after image reconstruction) for dual-source DE acquisitions because of the noncoincidence of projection data [1].

A wider range of monochromatic energies is available for each DE acquisition. For example, a DE acquisition at 80 and 140 kV can produce monochromatic images from 40 to 190 keV [2]. Monochromatic images characteristically exhibit less beam hardening artifacts than polychromatic images. Virtual images reconstructed at different monochromatic energy levels result in differences in image noise and iodine enhancement characteristics (Fig. 3.1), and reconstruction at an optimum monochromatic level theoretically improves image quality, tumor enhancement, and contrast-to-noise ratio [1, 3]. In a study on head and neck squamous cell carcinoma (SCC), reconstruction of monochromatic virtual images at 60 keV was found to result in improvement of subjective image quality, higher tumor attenuation, and increased tumor contrast-to-noise ratio [4].

3.3   Linear Image Blending

The low- and high-energy datasets of DE acquisition differ in their image properties. The low-energy image dataset is characterized by higher attenuation of iodinated contrast material as result of greater photoelectric effect and decreased Compton scattering at lower tube voltage. On the other, image noise will also increase. The high-energy image dataset is characterized by low image noise but at the expense of a lower attenuation of contrast material [5].

Mixed or blended image datasets could be readily reconstructed from the low- and high-energy acquisitions. The weighting factor or the blending ratio determines the contribution of low- and high-energy acquisition into the blended image dataset

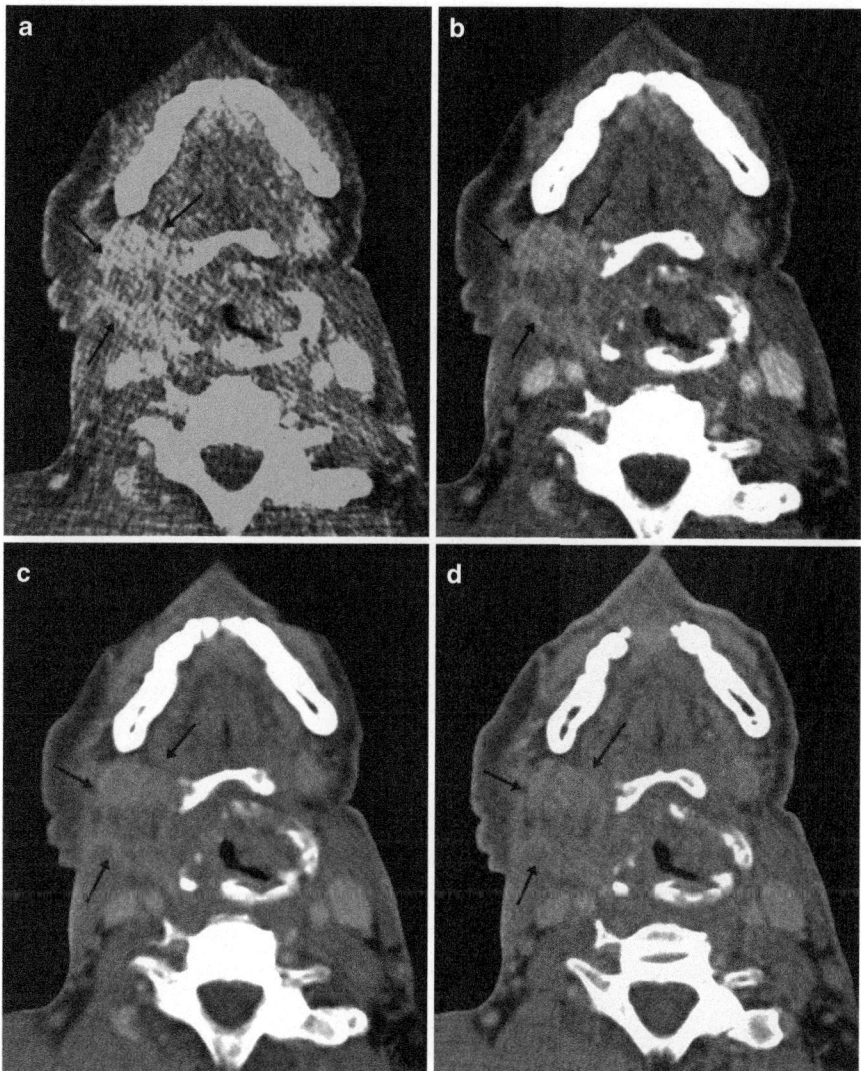

Fig. 3.1 Virtual monochromatic energies. (**a**) CT image reconstructed at 40 kev. (**b**) CT image reconstructed at 60 keV (**c**) CT image reconstructed at 80 keV. (**d**) Average weighted image used for routine clinical diagnosis. The lesion delineation (*arrows*) and image quality are optimized at 60 keV

(Fig. 3.2). In practice, a single linear blended image dataset is routinely reconstructed for clinical use. At tube voltages 80 and 140 kVp, the 0.3 blending ratio (30 % from 80 kVp data and 70 % from 140 kVp data) is used to reproduce the image quality of a conventional single-energy 120-kVp acquisition [6]. Blended images are potentially superior to conventional single-energy images because the total radiation dose of the DECT acquisition is utilized, thus reducing quantum noise.

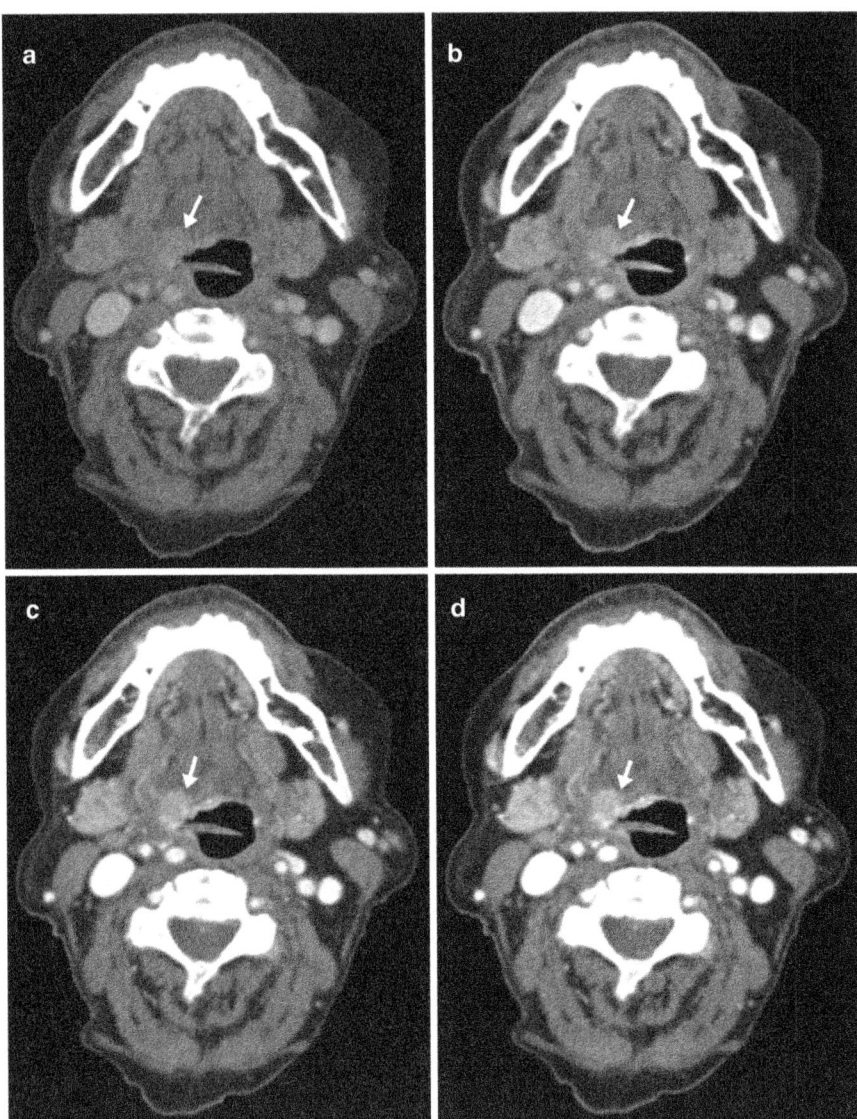

Fig. 3.2 Linear image blending. (**a**) 140-kVp image. (**b**) 0.3 weighted-average image (30 % from 80 kVp and 70 % from 140 kVp). (**c**) 0.6 weighted-average image (60 % from 80 kVp). (**d**) 0.8 weighted-average image (80 % from 80 kVp). (**e**) 80-kVp image. The lesion (*arrow*) and vascular contrast enhancement increase gradually as the tube energy is lowered from (**a**) through (**b**). Image noise also increases

Fig. 3.2 (continued)

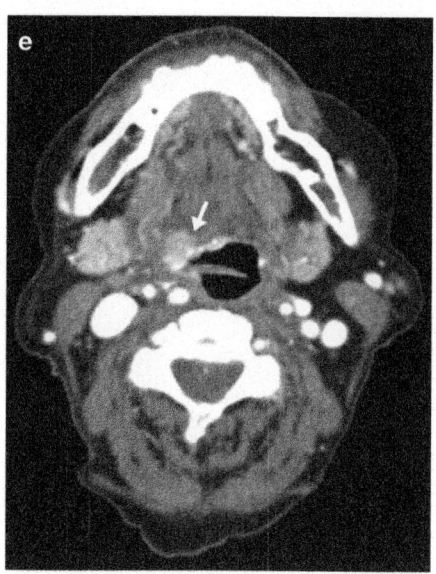

   Manual manipulation of the blending ratio may be attempted to generate different datasets with variable high contrast contribution from lower energy dataset and low noise level from higher energy dataset, until the best image quality and contrast for an individual scan is reached. This method is, unfortunately, time consuming and can only be done on dedicated workstation. A more practical approach is that a single image dataset with predetermined blending ratio is to be reconstructed and sent to the PACS at the time of CT acquisition. A preliminary study on SCC of the upper aerodigestive tract has reported improved image quality, contrast-to-noise ratios, and subjective lesion delineation using a blending ratio of 0.6 (60 % from 80 kVp and 40 % from Sn140 kVp) compared to the conventional 0.3 blending ratio [7].

3.4   Nonlinear Image Blending

Linear blending of low- and high-energy data uses the same mixing ratio across all the pixels of the image. Alternatively, another approach, nonlinear blending, was developed to increase contrast and minimize noise in the image. Nonlinear blending calculates a different mixing ratio for each image pixel according to a specific formula, depending on the attenuation value of the pixel as a variable. Several nonlinear blending functions have been developed, including binary blending, slope blending, Gaussian, modified sigmoid, and piecewise functions [8]. With nonlinear blending, pixels with attenuation are weighted preferentially towards low-energy data to maximize iodine contrast, while pixels with low attenuation are weighted towards the high-energy data to minimize image noise.

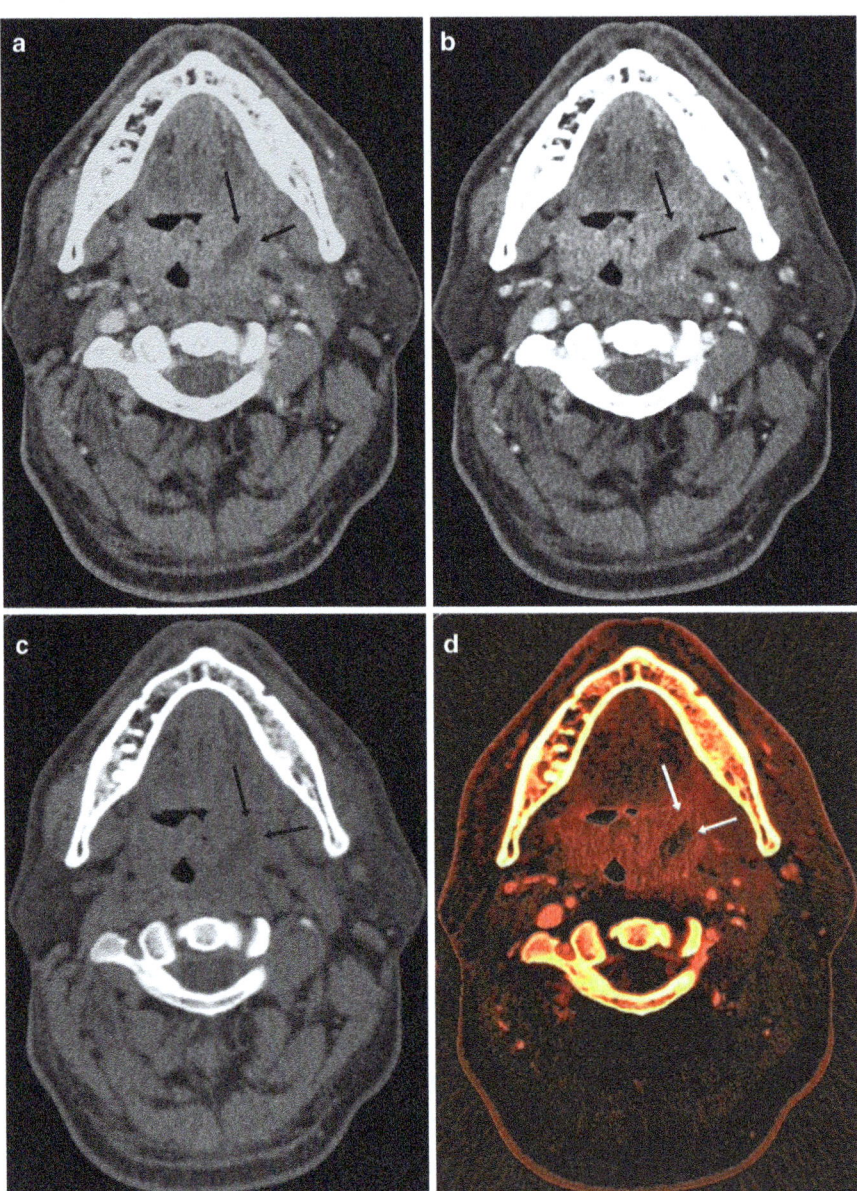

Fig. 3.3 Nonlinear image blending. Virtual unenhanced image. Iodine map. (**a**) Axial CT image showing an enhancing left tonsillar lesion with central necrosis (*arrows*). (**b**) Nonlinear blended image showing high contrast enhancement in the lesion (*arrows*) with low image noise and improved image quality. (**c**) Virtual unenhanced image. (**d**) Iodine map with iodine color code superimposed on the virtual unenhanced image

Nonlinear blending results in improved contrast-to-noise values and improved image quality compared to linear blending methods [9] (Fig. 3.3). A study on the use of nonlinear blending in imaging of oral carcinoma reported high contrast and low noise and hence high lesion signal-to-noise ratio and potential improvement in delineation of oral carcinoma [10]. Optimization of nonblending methods in DECT imaging of different body regions is an interesting subject of research [11, 12].

3.5   Iodine Distribution Map

DE scanning allows material decomposition so that iodine could be differentiated from soft tissue in a contrast-enhanced scan. The approach to iodine characterization differs slightly between single-source and dual-source DECT. Single-source DECT utilizes a two-material decomposition algorithm in the projection (raw data) domain. The attenuation values of the two selected base materials (e.g., water and iodine) at low and high energies are used to generate iodine images and virtual unenhanced images. With dual-source DECT, a three-material decomposition algorithm is utilized in the image domain (after image reconstruction), and is based on the differences in attenuation properties of three materials (e.g., iodine, soft tissue, and fat) at low and high energies. Iodine images and virtual unenhanced images could be then generated [13].

Iodine images may be displayed as gray-scale images or as color-coded overlay maps (Fig. 3.3). In head and neck oncologic imaging, the color-coded map is thought to increase visual lesion detection. Because color is superimposed on original CT images, excellent anatomic details are preserved. Enhanced tumor tissue (color-coded because of iodine content) could be differentiated from other nonenhanced or noniodine containing tissue, even if the CT attenuation values were similar. One of the advantages of iodine overlay maps is the improved depiction of cartilage invasion by hypopharyngeal and laryngeal SCC. In a study by Kuno et al., the addition of color-coded iodine maps to the CT examination of SCC improved the accuracy of diagnosis of cartilage invasion. Iodine maps resulted in improved visual differentiation between the enhanced color-coded tumor and the unenhanced noncalcified thyroid cartilage, thus resulting in higher specificity and diagnostic confidence [14].

Virtual unenhanced images enable differentiation of enhanced lesions from calcification or other high attenuation lesions, without the necessity of scanning the patient before contrast administration.

3.6   Iodine Quantification

The degree of contrast uptake is calculated on conventional CT imaging by double scanning before and after contrast material administration and then subtracting unenhanced from enhanced attenuation values. With DECT, virtual unenhanced images may be used instead of true unenhanced images, thus eliminating the need

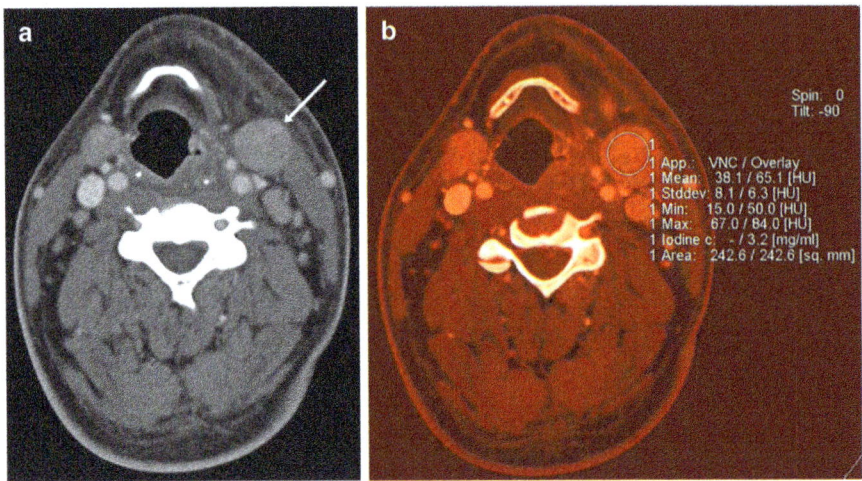

Fig. 3.4 Iodine quantification. (**a**) Axial CT image in a patient with bilateral enlarged deep cervical lymph nodes, the largest on the left side (*arrow*). (**b**) Axial iodine map at the same level showing iodine quantification in the enlarged left deep cervical lymph node (iodine overlay 65.1 HU and iodine content 3.2 mg/ml)

for scanning before contrast administration so that the patient's radiation exposure is nearly halved. Another advantage of DE technique is that calculations are performed with single ROI insertion so that misregistration errors in ROI insertion between unenhanced and enhanced scans are avoided.

The contrast uptake in any given lesion is the difference between its attenuation on contrast-enhanced and (virtual) unenhanced images. This net iodine uptake is termed the "iodine overlay" (measured in HU). The utility of iodine overlay measurements in assessment of the degree of enhancement was found to be comparable to conventional CT measurements [15, 16].

Another new approach offered by DECT for calculation of the degree of contrast uptake is termed the "iodine content," measured in mg/ml (Fig. 3.4). Iodine content is calculated by detection of the presence of iodine itself and the direct quantification of iodine in each voxel using the three-material decomposition algorithm [17]. Iodine content quantification was found to be at least as accurate as standard enhancement measurements in distinguishing enhancing from nonenhancing masses [18, 19].

Pathophysiologic changes that affect tissue microvascularity, such as tumor-related neoangiogenesis, which leads to increased regional blood volume and capillary hyperpermeability, result in a higher degree of contrast enhancement on CT [20]. Assessment of the degree of contrast uptake by soft tissue tumors may help in tumor grading, differentiation between benign and malignant tumors, or between tumor recurrence and post-therapeutic changes.

Initial experience on the use of iodine content and iodine overlay measurements in the head and neck region demonstrated feasibility and simplicity of this method.

Preliminary results reported a promising role of DE, especially iodine content quantification method, in characterization of cervical lymphadenopathy [21].

3.7 Dual Energy CT in Brain Tumors

Studies investigating the use of DECT in imaging of primary or metastatic brain tumors are limited because MRI, rather than CT, is usually the modality of choice for brain imaging. Meanwhile, CT is the modality of choice in imaging of intracerebral hemorrhage. Detection of an underlying tumor as the cause of intracerebral hemorrhage is crucial, but sometimes difficult; because tumor enhancement may be masked by the high attenuation of hemorrhage. DECT can be useful in differentiation of iodine (tumor enhancement) from hemorrhage, and preliminary results on the clinical utility of DECT in detection of underlying brain tumors in intracerebral hemorrhage reported higher accuracy of DE-derived color-coded iodine images and virtual unenhanced images in detection of tumor enhancement compared to conventional post-contrast CT [22].

References

1. Yu L, Leng S, McCollough CH (2012) Dual-energy CT-based monochromatic imaging. AJR Am J Roentgenol 199(5 Suppl):9–15
2. Yu L, Christner JA, Leng S, Wang J, Fletcher JG, McCollough CH (2011) Virtual monochromatic imaging in dual-source dual-energy CT: radiation dose and image quality. Med Phys 38:6371–6379
3. Pomerantz SR, Kamalian S, Zhang D, Gupta R, Rapalino O, Sahani DV, Lev MH (2013) Virtual monochromatic reconstruction of dual-energy unenhanced head CT at 65–75 keV maximizes image quality compared with conventional polychromatic CT. Radiology 266:318–325
4. Wichmann JL, Nöske EM, Kraft J, Burck I, Wagenblast J, Eckardt A, Frellesen C, Kerl JM, Bauer RW, Bodelle B, Lehnert T, Vogl TJ, Schulz B (2014) Virtual monoenergetic dual-energy computed tomography: optimization of kiloelectron volt settings in head and neck cancer. Invest Radiol 49:735–741
5. Vogl TJ, Schulz B, Bauer RW, Stöver T, Sader R, Tawfik AM (2012) Dual-energy CT applications in head and neck imaging. AJR Am J Roentgenol 199(5 Suppl):S34–S39
6. Tawfik AM, Kerl JM, Razek AA et al (2011) Image quality and radiation dose of dual-energy CT of the head and neck compared with a standard 120-kVp acquisition. AJNR Am J Neuroradiol 32:1994–1999
7. Tawfik AM, Kerl JM, Bauer RW et al (2012) Dual-energy CT of head and neck cancer: average weighting of low- and high-voltage acquisitions to improve lesion delineation and image quality-initial clinical experience. Invest Radiol 47:306–311
8. Marin D, Boll DT, Mileto A, Nelson RC (2014) State of the art: dual-energy CT of the abdomen. Radiology 271:327–342
9. Ascenti G, Krauss B, Mazziotti S, Mileto A, Settineri N, Vinci S, Donato R, Gaeta M (2012) Dual-energy computed tomography (DECT) in renal masses: nonlinear versus linear blending. Acad Radiol 19:1186–1193

10. Toepker M, Czerny C, Ringl H, Fruehwald-Pallamar J, Wolf F, Weber M, Ploder O, Klug C (2014) Can dual-energy CT improve the assessment of tumor margins in oral cancer? Oral Oncol 50:221–227
11. Kim KS, Lee JM, Kim SH et al (2010) Image fusion in dual energy computed tomography for detection of hypervascular liver hepatocellular carcinoma: phantom and preliminary studies. Invest Radiol 45:149–157
12. Lv P, Liu J, Wu R, Hou P, Hu L, Gao J (2014) Use of non-linear image blending with dual-energy CT improves vascular visualization in abdominal angiography. Clin Radiol 69:93–99
13. Agrawal MD, Pinho DF, Kulkarni NM, Hahn PF, Guimaraes AR, Sahani DV (2014) Oncologic applications of dual-energy CT in the abdomen. Radiographics 34:589–612
14. Kuno H, Onaya H, Iwata R, Kobayashi T, Fujii S, Hayashi R, Otani K, Ojiri H, Yamanaka T, Satake M (2012) Evaluation of cartilage invasion by laryngeal and hypopharyngeal squamous cell carcinoma with dual-energy CT. Radiology 265:488–496
15. Chae EJ, Song JW, Seo JB, Krauss B, Jang YM, Song KS (2008) Clinical utility of dual-energy CT in the evaluation of solitary pulmonary nodules: initial experience. Radiology 249:671–681
16. Song KD, Kim CK, Park BK, Kim B (2011) Utility of iodine overlay technique and virtual unenhanced images for the characterization of renal masses by dual-energy CT. AJR Am J Roentgenol 197:1076–1082
17. Chandarana H, Megibow AJ, Cohen BA et al (2011) Iodine quantification with dual-energy CT: phantom study and preliminary experience with renal masses. AJR Am J Roentgenol 196:693–700
18. Ascenti G, Mileto A, Krauss B et al (2013) Distinguishing enhancing from nonenhancing renal masses with dual-source dual energy CT: iodine quantification versus standard enhancement measurements. Eur Radiol 23:2288–2295
19. Mileto A, Marin D, Ramirez-Giraldo JC, Scribano E, Krauss B, Mazziotti S, Ascenti G (2014) Accuracy of contrast-enhanced dual-energy MDCT for the assessment of iodine uptake in renal lesions. AJR Am J Roentgenol 202:W466–W474
20. Miles KA (1999) Tumour angiogenesis and its relation to contrast enhancement on computed tomography: a review. Eur J Radiol 30:198–205
21. Tawfik AM, Razek AA, Kerl JM, Nour-Eldin NE, Bauer R, Vogl TJ (2014) Comparison of dual-energy CT-derived iodine content and iodine overlay of normal, inflammatory and metastatic squamous cell carcinoma cervical lymph nodes. Eur Radiol 24:574–580
22. Kim SJ, Lim HK, Lee HY, Choi CG, Lee DH, Suh DC, Kim SM, Kim JK, Krauss B (2012) Dual-energy CT in the evaluation of intracerebral hemorrhage of unknown origin: differentiation between tumor bleeding and pure hemorrhage. AJNR Am J Neuroradiol 33:865–872

Dual Energy CT in Chest Tumors

4

Felix G. Meinel, Long Jiang Zhang, and U. Joseph Schoepf

4.1   Introduction

The promise of dual energy computed tomography (DECT) of the chest is to add functional information to the anatomical depiction of the thoracic organs. This possibility has been investigated in a variety of oncologic applications (Table 4.1). Iodine uptake has been used to characterize pulmonary nodules as benign or malignant and to assess the viability and therapy response of thoracic tumors. DECT-derived maps of iodine distribution in the pulmonary parenchyma can be used as a surrogate for pulmonary perfusion, which may be of particular interest in the preoperative evaluation of patients with lung cancer and in the assessment of pulmonary embolism as a common complication of malignancies. Noble gases such as Xenon can be used to visualize pulmonary ventilation. Finally, the spectral information from DECT data enables novel postprocessing algorithms that can improve the contrast-to-noise characteristics of chest CT. In this chapter, we aim to provide an overview over the possible ways DECT has been used for oncologic imaging of the chest and its utility in these applications.

F.G. Meinel (✉)
Institute for Clinical Radiology, Ludwig-Maximilians-University Hospital,
Marchioninistr. 15, Munich 81377, Germany
e-mail: felix.meinel@med.lmu.de

L.J. Zhang
Department of Medical Imaging, Jinling Hospital, Medical School of Nanjing University,
305 Zhongshan Easr Road, Nanjing, Jiangsu Province 210002, China
e-mail: kevinzhlj@163.com

U.J. Schoepf
Department of Radiology and Radiological Science, Medical University
of South Carolina, 25 Courtenay Drive, Charleston, SC 29425, USA
e-mail: schoepf@musc.edu

© Springer International Publishing Switzerland 2015
C.N. De Cecco et al. (eds.), *Dual Energy CT in Oncology*,
DOI 10.1007/978-3-319-19563-6_4

Table 4.1 Oncologic applications of dual energy chest CT

Characterization of lung nodules/masses as benign or malignant
Imaging in confirmed lung cancer
Assessment of tumor vitality and therapy response
Nodal staging
Imaging pulmonary embolism in cancer patients
Pulmonary perfusion imaging
Pulmonary ventilation imaging
Optimization of image contrast
Monoenergetic extrapolation
Nonlinear blending techniques

4.2   Assessment of Lung Nodules and Thoracic Malignancies

4.2.1   Acquisition Technique

DECT of the thorax can be performed using either single-source CT systems equipped with a rapid kV switching X-ray tube or dual source CT systems. With dual source CT systems, DECT is performed analogous to a conventional contrast-enhanced chest CT except that the tube current is distributed over both tubes, which are operated at different photon energies. The recommended spectral combination differs between the various generations of CT systems with the lower energy spectrum ranging from 80 to 100 kVp and the higher energy spectrum ranging from 140 to 150 kVp. In the more recent generations of dual source CT systems, the higher energy spectrum can be hardened by means of a tin filter in order to decrease the overlap in photon energies between both spectra. If the goal of performing DECT is the assessment of lung nodules, masses or lymph nodes, the examination is typically acquired in a venous phase to ensure adequate contrast enhancement of these structures although an arterial phase may be added depending on the clinical indication. In the delayed phase, the enhancement of the pulmonary parenchyma is minimal. If an assessment of pulmonary perfusion is desired, an additional dual energy CT pulmonary angiography (DE-CTPA) needs to be acquired, as described in more detail below.

4.2.2   Characterization of Pulmonary Nodules/Masses as Benign or Malignant

Pulmonary nodules are frequently detected in chest CT. This includes CT staging examinations in patients with extra-thoracic malignancies, incidentally detected nodules in patients without an underlying oncologic diagnosis or nodules detected at lung cancer screening. The latter two scenarios are particularly challenging, since the pre-test probability of malignancy is relatively low. Several clinical risk factors as well as nodule size and characteristics have been shown to predict the likelihood of malignancy [1, 2]. Nevertheless, for an individual patient, these clues are often not sufficient to classify a nodule as either clearly benign or malignant. In this context, the ability of DECT to visualize and quantify the iodine uptake of pulmonary nodules has been explored as a means to differentiate benign from malignant pulmonary nodules [3]. DECT examples of malignant and benign pulmonary masses are shown in Figs. 4.1, 4.2, 4.3, 4.4, and 4.5, respectively. Chae and colleagues [4] evaluated the clinical utility of DECT for the classification of 45 solitary pulmonary nodules, which were confirmed as benign or malignant on the basis of percutaneous needle aspiration histology. In their study, the diagnostic accuracy for malignancy by using CT numbers on iodine-enhanced image series with a cutoff of 20 HU was comparable to that achieved by using the degree of enhancement. More recently, Hou and colleagues [5] compared the dual energy CT characteristics of 35 patients with lung cancers to those of 25 patients with inflammatory masses using a dual phase (arterial and venous phase) CT acquisition protocol. They found significant differences in iodine uptake between both groups. The iodine content in the center of masses in the venous acquisition phase (normalized to the aorta) had the highest discriminatory power with lower central iodine content in lung cancers compared to inflammatory masses. Kawai and colleagues [6] evaluated the feasibility of measuring iodine uptake of ground glass lesions by DECT. This study provided preliminary data that iodine uptake may be useful for the characterization of ground glass opacities as they found an increased iodine-related attenuation in adenocarcinomas compared to pulmonary hemorrhage or inflammatory changes. The presence and pattern of calcifications of lung nodules is another important feature that can suggest a benign or malignant entity. Virtual noncontrast images can be reconstructed from DECT data and have been found useful in differentiating iodine enhancement from calcifications in lung nodules (Figs. 4.2 and 4.3) [7].

4.2.3   Lung Cancer: Assessment of Tumor Perfusion, Therapy Response, and Staging

The assessment of patients with a confirmed diagnosis of lung cancer represents a very different scenario. Here, the potential utility of DECT could be to assess tumor vitality and response to therapy. In addition, visualization of iodine uptake has been explored as a tool for the visualization and characterization of mediastinal lymph nodes in the nodal staging of lung cancer (Fig. 4.1). Schmid-Bindert and colleagues [8] have demonstrated that the iodine uptake of non-small cell lung cancers measured by DECT correlates with metabolic activity on FDG-PET. The correlation between metabolic activity at PET and the iodine-related attenuation at DECT was lower for thoracic lymph nodes compared to the primary tumor [8]. In a pilot study of ten patients with non-small cell lung cancer treated with the anti-angiogenic agent Bevacizumab, Kim and colleagues used DECT-derived tumor enhancement to assess therapy response [9]. In their study, the spectral information from DECT was considered particularly useful to discriminate between tumor enhancement and

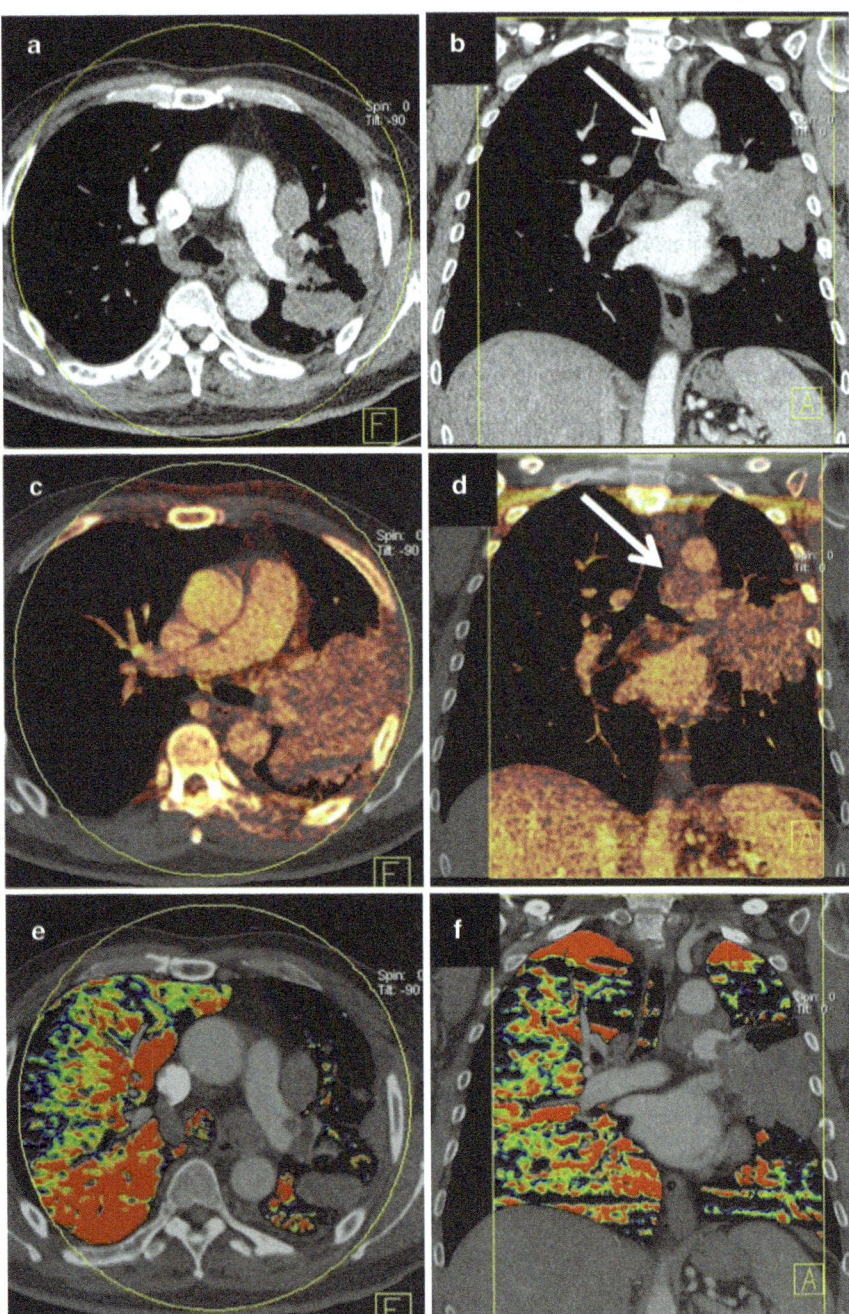

Fig. 4.1 Dual energy CT in a 56-year-old male patient with squamous cell lung cancer. Average weighted reconstructions in the arterial phase in axial and coronal orientation (**a**, **b**) demonstrate a large, left-sided pulmonary mass with infiltration of the left main pulmonary artery. The iodine overlay images from the venous acquisition phase (**c**, **d**) demonstrate strong, relatively homogeneous perfusion of the tumor. Iodine uptake of mediastinal lymph node metastasis is also noted. Iodine distribution maps derived from dual energy CT pulmonary angiography (**e**, **f**) demonstrate substantially decreased perfusion to the entire left lung due to obstruction of the left main pulmonary artery

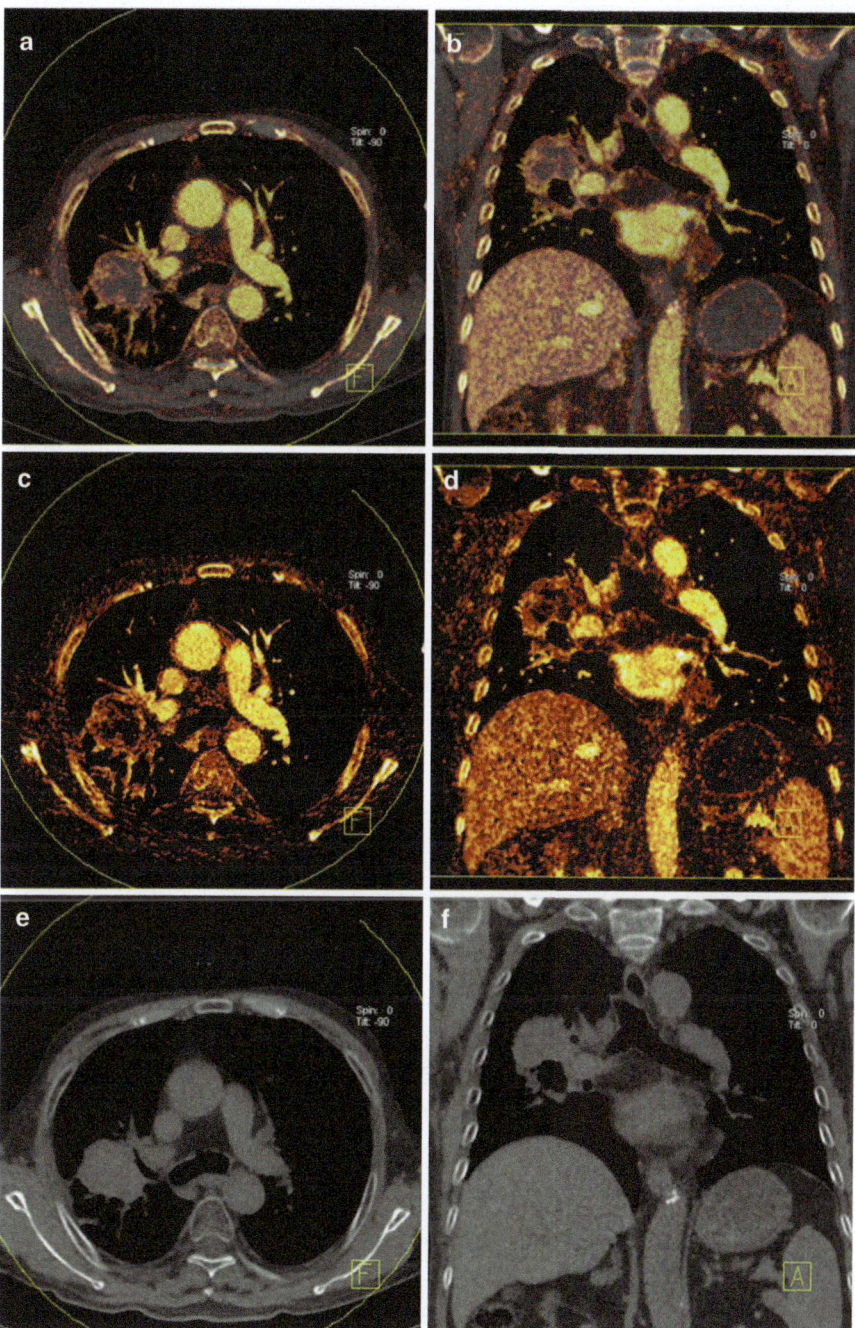

Fig. 4.2 Dual energy CT in an 83-year-old male patient with non-small cell lung cancer. Iodine overlay images (**a**, **b**) and pure iodine images (**c**, **d**) demonstrate strong perfusion in the periphery of the tumor and low perfusion in its necrotic center. Virtual noncontrast images (**e**, **f**) demonstrate absence of calcification within the mass

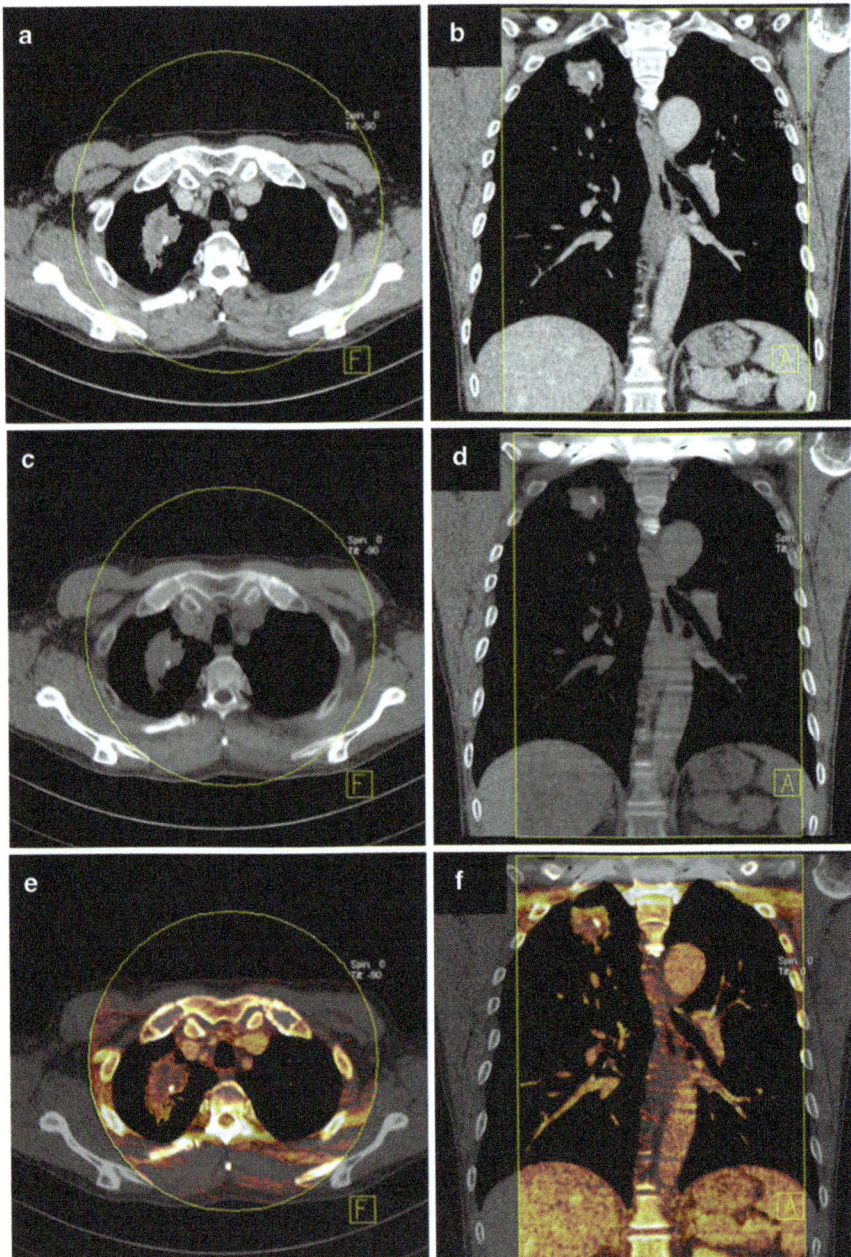

Fig. 4.3 Dual energy CT in a 63-year-old male patient with adenocarcinoma in the right upper lobe. Average weighted reconstructions in the venous phase in axial and coronal orientation (**a, b**) demonstrate a mass in the right upper lobe. Virtual noncontrast reconstructions (**c, d**) demonstrate a small calcification within the mass. Iodine overlay images (**e, f**) demonstrate strong iodine uptake, particularly in the periphery of the mass

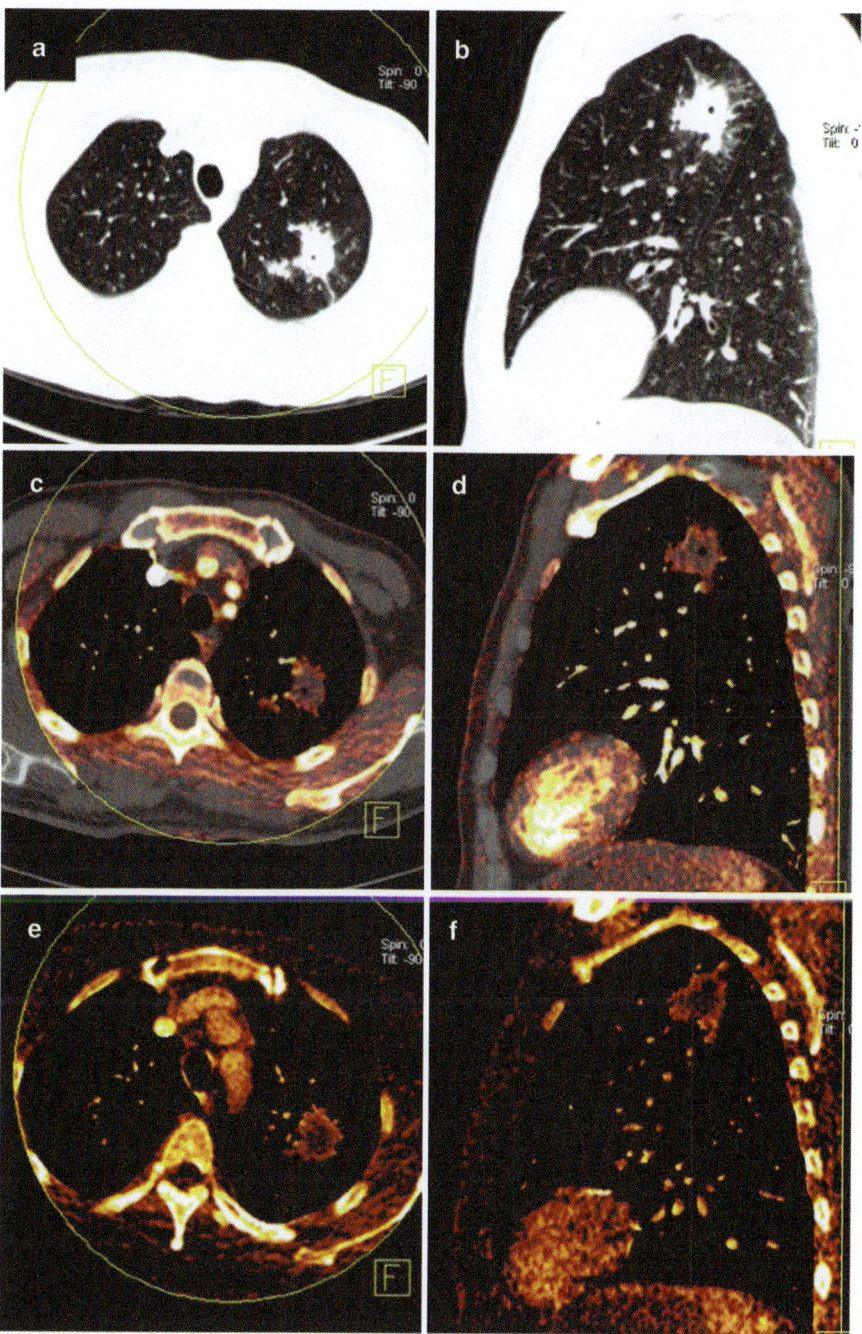

Fig. 4.4 Dual energy CT in a 52-year-old male patient with tuberculosis. Average weighted reconstructions displayed in a lung window in axial and sagittal orientation (**a**, **b**) demonstrate a large mass with spiculated margins in the left upper lobe. Iodine overlay images in the arterial phase (**c**, **d**) and pure iodine images in the venous phase (**e**, **f**) demonstrate rim-like iodine uptake in the periphery of the mass

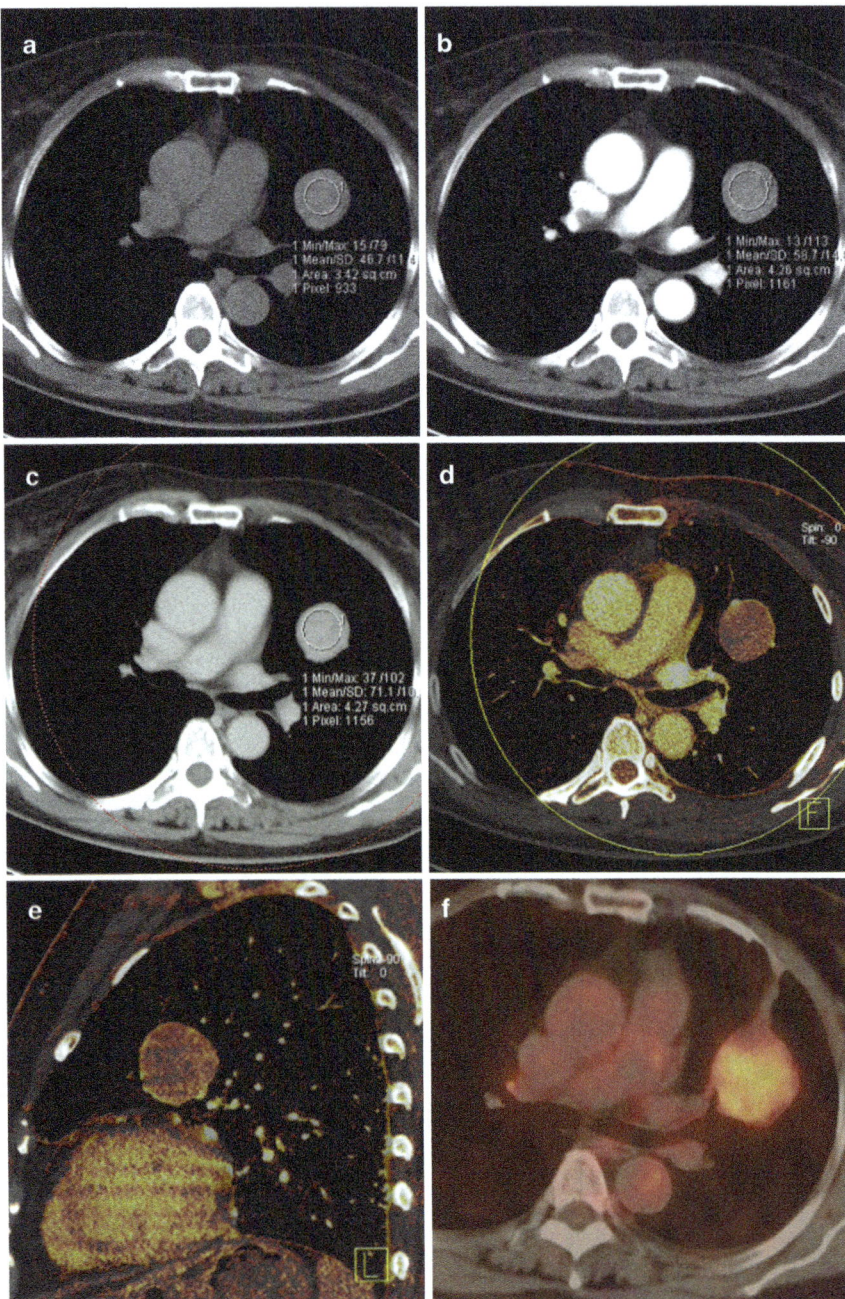

Fig. 4.5 Dual energy CT in a 61-year-old female patient with a sclerosing hemangioma of the lung. The mass is shown on axial average weighted CTPA reconstructions in noncontrast (**a**), arterial (**b**) and venous phase (**c**). The perfusion of the mass is assessed using dual energy iodine distribution maps in the venous acquisition phase shown in axial and sagittal orientation (**d**, **e**). The corresponding 18 F-FDG-PET/CT image is shown in panel (**f**). Sclerosing hemangioma of the lung is an uncommon neoplasm. Although lymph node metastasis has been reported, sclerosing hemangioma is generally considered a benign lesion and surgical excision is curative [47]

intratumor hemorrhage. Baxa and colleagues [10] retrospectively analyzed the DECT characteristics of mediastinal lymph nodes in patients with non-small cell lung cancer who underwent dual phase (arterial and venous phase) DECT before and after chemotherapy. They noticed that enlarged lymph nodes showed a higher arterial enhancement fraction compared to nonenlarged lymph nodes. In lymph nodes shrinking under chemotherapy, a significant decrease in arterial enhancement fraction was observed.

4.2.4 Lung Cancer: Assessment of Pulmonary Perfusion and/or Ventilation

In patients with lung cancer, particular those with a centrally located tumor compromising the hilar vessels or bronchi, preoperative DECT has been used to predict postoperative pulmonary perfusion and ventilation. Chae and colleagues [11] found that DECT can predict postoperative lung function more accurately than scintigraphy. In their study, DECT was superior to scintigraphy for the depiction of perfusion and ventilation defects and assessing collateral ventilation in patients with centrally located lung cancers.

4.3 Lung Perfusion Imaging in Pulmonary Embolism

Dual energy CT pulmonary angiography (DE-CTPA) can visualize the iodine distribution within the pulmonary parenchyma as a surrogate for pulmonary perfusion [12–17]. The resulting iodine distribution maps have been validated against scintigraphy [18] and SPECT [19] images in clinical studies and against dynamic CT measurements of pulmonary perfusion in animal models [20]. The main application of dual energy lung perfusion imaging has been the diagnosis and assessment of pulmonary embolism (Figs. 4.6 and 4.7). As such, the technique is highly relevant to oncologic imaging, considering that malignancy is one the major risk factors for pulmonary embolism [21].

4.3.1 Acquisition Technique

System-specific recommendations for DE-CTPA acquisition parameters have been proposed in the literature [22]. Both test bolus or bolus tracking techniques can be used. A slightly longer delay (5–7 s) than for conventional CTPA is typically chosen to allow for the contrast material to reach the pulmonary capillary system. An iodine delivery rate of approximately 1.6 g I/s has been found to result in optimal image quality for both morphological CTPA reconstructions and dual energy perfusion maps [15]. In order to minimize streak artifacts originating from dense contrast material in the superior vena cava, some institutions prefer a triphasic injection protocol in which the contrast agent bolus is followed by 30 mL of a mixture of

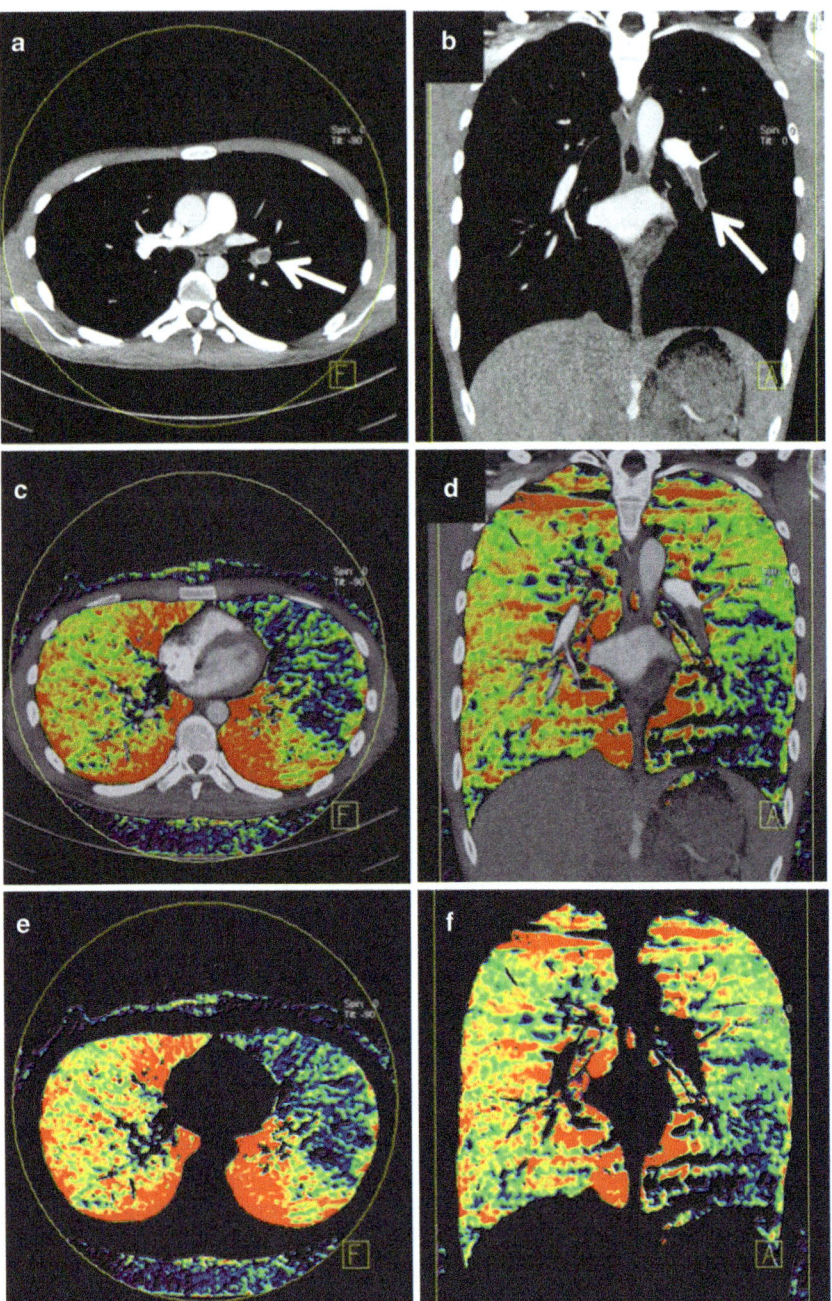

Fig. 4.6 Dual energy CTPA in a 28-year-old male patient with pulmonary embolism. CTPA in axial (**a**) and coronal (**b**) orientation demonstrates a filling defect in the left inferior pulmonary artery (*arrows*). Iodine overlay images (**c, d**) as well as pure iodine distribution maps (**e, f**) demonstrate a corresponding perfusion defect in the left lower lobe

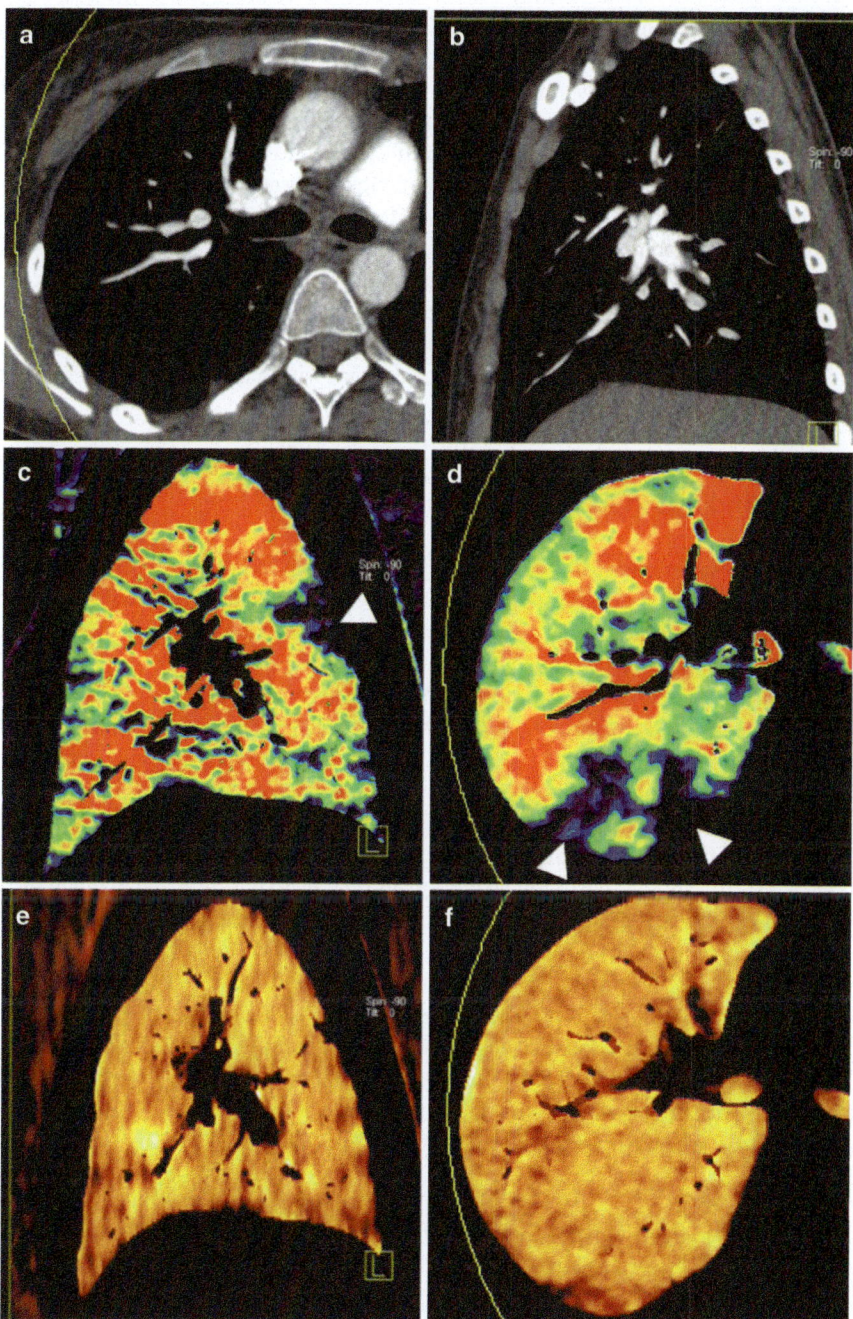

Fig. 4.7 Dual energy CTPA in a 19-year-old female patient with pulmonary embolism. Average weighted CTPA reconstructions in axial (**a**) and sagittal (**b**) orientation do not conclusively demonstrate pulmonary emboli. However, dual energy iodine distribution maps (**c, d**) demonstrate multiple peripheral wedge-shaped perfusion defects (*arrowheads*) suggesting subsegmental pulmonary embolism. Xenon distribution maps (**e, f**) demonstrate homogeneous ventilation and thus mismatch of ventilation and perfusion findings

saline and contrast agent, followed by a 50 mL saline chaser [23]. Choosing a cau-docranial direction of acquisition further helps minimize artifacts from dense contrast material in the superior vena cava. As with conventional CTPA, deep inspiration prior to breathhold should be avoided, since the inflow of nonopacified blood from the inferior vena cava during deep inspiration can lead to an interruption of the contrast bolus and inadequate opacification of the pulmonary circulation. From the acquired low- and high-energy datasets, anatomical image series similar to a conventional CTPA can be reconstructed by mixing the data from both energy levels. In addition, specific postprocessing software is used to segment the pulmonary parenchyma and then display pulmonary iodine content as a color-coded parametric map (Figs. 4.6 and 4.7). By means of a different postprocessing algorithm, DE-CTPA data can also be used to visualize the iodine content within the pulmonary vessels to increase the conspicuity of emboli [24].

4.3.2   Findings in Acute Pulmonary Embolism

Iodine distribution maps of the pulmonary parenchyma in patients with pulmonary embolism typically demonstrate wedge-shaped, peripherally located areas of decreased iodine content, which follow a segmental or lobar anatomical distribution (Figs. 4.6 and 4.7) [22]. Animal studies [25] have concluded that the use of DECT iodine distribution maps may improve the sensitivity of CTPA, in particular for peripheral subsegmental emboli, but this has not been conclusively demonstrated in clinical studies. If DE-CTPA is routinely performed in patients with suspected pulmonary embolism, it is not uncommon to see one or more small peripheral perfusion defects with a pattern suggestive of embolic disease in patients in whom no intravascular filing defects are visualized on the morphological CT reconstructions (Fig. 4.7) [26]. There is currently no consensus on how to interpret and manage such cases [22]. If a reader with ample experience in interpreting DE-CTPA cannot explain them by artifacts or other pathology, such perfusion defects likely represent subsegmental emboli too small to be visualized anatomically and should be mentioned in the radiology report as suspicious for small, subsegmental emboli. DE-CTPA datasets also enable automated quantification of pulmonary perfused blood volume. The values of pulmonary perfused blood volume have been shown to inversely correlate with the severity of acute pulmonary embolism [27–29] and may carry adverse prognostic significance in this setting [28, 30, 31].

4.3.3   Caveats and Pitfalls in the Interpretation of Dual Energy Lung Perfusion Maps

The interpretation of DE-CTPA lung perfusion maps can be challenging. In particular, experience is required to confidently distinguish artifacts from true perfusion defects [32] and to differentiate between perfusion defects related to pulmonary embolism and defects caused by other pathologies [33]. To minimize misinterpretation errors, the visual analysis of DECT lung perfusion maps should be performed in side-by-side correlation with the anatomical reconstruction series. This will allow readers to directly correlate perfusion defects with vascular territories and segmental anatomy and to match anatomical changes of the pulmonary parenchyma with alterations in the perfusion maps.

In addition, the influence of several technical and physiological factors should be considered. Pulmonary iodine distribution (perfusion) maps are generated based on a single CTPA acquisition and thus visualize the iodine distribution in the pulmonary capillary circulation at this one specific time point – which is regarded as a surrogate for pulmonary perfusion. Due to the inherent limitations of such a single-shot technique, the iodine content within the pulmonary microcirculation is influenced by a multitude of technical and physiological parameters. The timing of the scan relative to the contrast bolus plays an important role [34]. One should also be aware that the CT acquisition is timed to ensure optimal contrast enhancement of the pulmonary capillary system. The "perfusion" maps derived from DE-CTPA acquisitions thus primarily visualize lung perfusion from the pulmonary circulation and neglect contributions from the systemic circulation. The concentration, volume, delivery rate of the administered contrast agent, and interindividual physiologic differences further influence pulmonary parenchymal enhancement at the time of image acquisition. Furthermore, lung density physiologically decreases with age [35], leading to a decrease in pulmonary parenchymal iodine uptake on DECT perfusion maps with older age even in the absence of pathology [34].

4.4   Ventilation Imaging in Pulmonary Embolism

Dual energy CT has been explored for imaging pulmonary ventilation. This requires the administration of radiopaque noble gases (most commonly, Xenon) as inhalative contrast agents. The unique potential of ventilation CT is its ability to visualize the spatial distribution of pathologic ventilation patterns, which are not accessible to conventional CT imaging or pulmonary function tests. However, Xenon-enhanced DECT has never been widely adopted in clinical routine, mostly because the procedure is technically very challenging [36]. In addition, Xenon is not routinely available, expensive, and can have potentially severe side effects including respiratory depression [16, 37, 38].

4.4.1   Acquisition Technique

Xenon-enhanced ventilation CT requires careful patient preparation and monitoring. Patients are fitted with ventilation masks, unless they are mechanically ventilated. Respiratory rate, oxygen saturation and blood pressure, inspirational and expirational concentrations of Xenon are continuously monitored before, during, and after the CT examination. After applying a high oxygen fraction (>60 %) for approximately 2–3 min, a mixture of 30 % Xenon and 70 % oxygen is administered.

During the wash-in phase, which typically lasts around 60–90 s, normally ventilated lung areas are saturated with Xenon. When the exhaled Xenon concentration reaches approximately 30 %, the patient returns to inhaling highly concentrated oxygen for an approximately 2 min wash-out phase until the expiratory Xenon concentration approaches zero. CT images are typically acquired at a single time point at the end of the wash-in phase when normal lung areas are saturated with Xenon. The pulmonary Xenon distribution at this time point is captured as a surrogate for pulmonary ventilation.

4.4.2   Findings in Pulmonary Embolism

In patients with pulmonary embolism, combined ventilation/perfusion CT has been performed using intravenous iodine and inhaled Xenon as contrast agents. In this setting, CT can demonstrate ventilation/perfusion mismatch (Fig. 4.7) [39, 40].

4.5   Optimization of Image Properties Using Dual Energy–based Postprocessing

Acquiring data with two different spectra offers additional possibilities for postprocessing (Fig. 4.8). Based on the image characteristics with the two different spectra, virtual monoenergetic images can be generated, which simulate acquisition at specific photon energies. Extrapolation to high photon energies can reduce beam-hardening artifacts from metallic implants [41]. Virtual extrapolation to low photon energies improves iodine contrast and can thus decrease the required volume of contrast agent [42, 43]. Nonlinear blending techniques optimize image contrast by integrating the higher iodine contrast of the lower energy spectrum with the superior noise characteristics of the higher energy spectrum. Without increasing radiation dose, this approach can improve contrast-to-noise-ratio in chest CT [44].

4.6   Radiation Dose Considerations

The dose of dual energy contrast-enhanced chest CT or dual energy CT pulmonary angiography typically falls in the range of 2.5–5 mSv with dual source CT systems [3, 26, 28, 40] and is thus comparable to the radiation dose associated with single energy CT at 120 kV using state-of-the-art CT equipment [7, 26, 44, 45]. However, dual energy acquisition for CT pulmonary angiography is incommensurable with novel dose-lowering techniques such as high-pitch or low kV acquisition. In patients suitable for these techniques, dual energy acquisition therefore requires a higher radiation dose. The estimated cancer risk associated with a single chest CT examination, if any, is low [46]. This is particularly true when imaging patients with a confirmed diagnosis of malignancy, which is much more likely to become

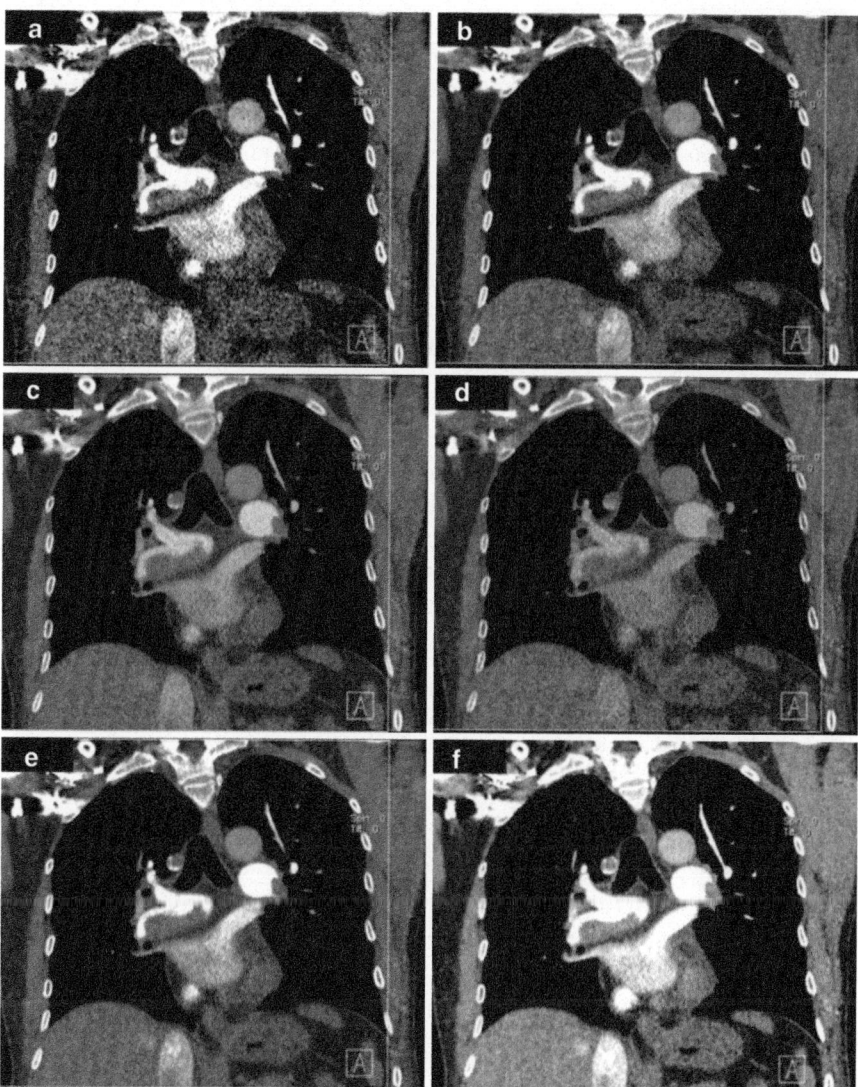

Fig. 4.8 Dual energy CTPA in a 48-year-old male patient with pulmonary embolism. Virtual monoenergetic images are shown extrapolated to photon energies of 50 keV (**a**), 60 keV (**b**), 80 keV (**c**), and 100 keV (**d**). Intravascular attenuation and image noise increase at low virtual photon energies. The optimal contrast image (**e**) generated with nonlinear blending techniques provides superior contrast-to-noise characteristics compared with the conventional average weighted image (**f**)

life-limiting for the patient. Nevertheless, CT examinations should only be acquired in dual energy acquisition mode if additional diagnostic information with a potential impact on patient management can reasonably be expected from the spectral information.

Conclusions

Dual energy chest CT has been explored in a variety of oncologic applications. Evidence regarding the utility of DECT for the characterization of lung nodules, nodal staging, and response assessment of lung cancer is scarce and limited to relatively small feasibility studies. The results were mixed and do not clearly show an incremental diagnostic value of DECT for these applications. Reliable data from well-designed studies on the value of the technique for clinical decision-making in oncologic patients is missing. Based on the currently available evidence, dual energy CT cannot be recommended for lung nodule characterization or tumor viability assessment outside of clinical studies. The use of DE-CTPA for visualization of pulmonary perfusion is fairly well validated and robust enough for clinical use. In cancer patients with pulmonary embolism or in the preoperative assessment of patients with lung cancer, DE-CTPA can be used to image lung perfusion, if this information carries potential significance for patient management. If chest CT is acquired in dual energy mode, dual energy–based postprocessing algorithms should be explored to enhance image quality.

References

1. McWilliams A et al (2013) Probability of cancer in pulmonary nodules detected on first screening CT. N Engl J Med 369(10):910–919
2. Horeweg N et al (2014) Lung cancer probability in patients with CT-detected pulmonary nodules: a prespecified analysis of data from the NELSON trial of low-dose CT screening. Lancet Oncol 15(12):1332–1341
3. Zhang LJ et al (2013) Dual-energy CT imaging of thoracic malignancies. Cancer Imaging 13:81–91
4. Chae EJ et al (2008) Clinical utility of dual-energy CT in the evaluation of solitary pulmonary nodules: initial experience. Radiology 249(2):671–681
5. Hou WS et al (2014) Differentiation of lung cancers from inflammatory masses with dual-energy spectral CT imaging. Acad Radiol 22(3):337–344
6. Kawai T et al (2011) Can dual-energy CT evaluate contrast enhancement of ground-glass attenuation? Phantom and preliminary clinical studies. Acad Radiol 18(6):682–689
7. Chae EJ et al (2010) Dual-energy computed tomography characterization of solitary pulmonary nodules. J Thorac Imaging 25(4):301–310
8. Schmid-Bindert G et al (2012) Functional imaging of lung cancer using dual energy CT: how does iodine related attenuation correlate with standardized uptake value of 18FDG-PET-CT? Eur Radiol 22(1):93–103
9. Kim YN et al (2012) Dual-energy CT in patients treated with anti-angiogenic agents for non-small cell lung cancer: new method of monitoring tumor response? Korean J Radiol 13(6):702–710
10. Baxa J et al (2014) Dual-phase dual-energy CT in patients with lung cancer: assessment of the additional value of iodine quantification in lymph node therapy response. Eur Radiol 24(8):1981–1988
11. Chae EJ et al (2013) Prediction of postoperative lung function in patients undergoing lung resection: dual-energy perfusion computed tomography versus perfusion scintigraphy. Invest Radiol 48(8):622–627
12. Thieme SF et al (2009) Dual-energy CT for the assessment of contrast material distribution in the pulmonary parenchyma. AJR Am J Roentgenol 193(1):144–149
13. Johnson TR et al (2007) Material differentiation by dual energy CT: initial experience. Eur Radiol 17(6):1510–1517

14. Lee CW et al (2012) A pilot trial on pulmonary emphysema quantification and perfusion mapping in a single-step using contrast-enhanced dual-energy computed tomography. Invest Radiol 47(1):92–97
15. Nance JW Jr et al (2012) Optimization of contrast material delivery for dual-energy computed tomography pulmonary angiography in patients with suspected pulmonary embolism. Invest Radiol 47(1):78–84
16. Remy-Jardin M et al (2010) Thoracic applications of dual energy. Radiol Clin North Am 48(1):193–205
17. Remy-Jardin M et al (2014) Thoracic applications of dual energy. Semin Respir Crit Care Med 35(1):64–73
18. Thieme SF et al (2008) Dual energy CT for the assessment of lung perfusion – correlation to scintigraphy. Eur J Radiol 68(3):369–374
19. Thieme SF et al (2012) Dual Energy CT lung perfusion imaging – correlation with SPECT/CT. Eur J Radiol 81(2):360–365
20. Fuld MK et al (2013) Pulmonary perfused blood volume with dual-energy CT as surrogate for pulmonary perfusion assessed with dynamic multidetector CT. Radiology 267(3):747–756
21. Goldhaber SZ (2010) Risk factors for venous thromboembolism. J Am Coll Cardiol 56(1):1–7
22. Lu GM et al (2012) Dual-energy CT of the lung. AJR Am J Roentgenol 199(5 Suppl):S40–S53
23. Kerl JM et al (2011) Triphasic contrast injection improves evaluation of dual energy lung perfusion in pulmonary CT angiography. Eur J Radiol 80(3):e483–e487
24. Tang CX et al (2013) Dual-energy CT based vascular iodine analysis improves sensitivity for peripheral pulmonary artery thrombus detection: an experimental study in canines. Eur J Radiol 82(12):2270–2278
25. Zhang LJ et al (2009) Pulmonary embolism detection with dual-energy CT: experimental study of dual-source CT in rabbits. Radiology 252(1):61–70
26. Pontana F et al (2008) Lung perfusion with dual-energy multidetector-row CT (MDCT): feasibility for the evaluation of acute pulmonary embolism in 117 consecutive patients. Acad Radiol 15(12):1494–1504
27. Nagayama H et al (2013) Quantification of lung perfusion blood volume (lung PBV) by dual-energy CT in pulmonary embolism before and after treatment: preliminary results. Clin Imaging 37(3):493–497
28. Meinel FG et al (2013) Effectiveness of automated quantification of pulmonary perfused blood volume using dual-energy CTPA for the severity assessment of acute pulmonary embolism. Invest Radiol 48(8):563–569
29. Sueyoshi E et al (2011) Quantification of lung perfusion blood volume (lung PBV) by dual-energy CT in patients with and without pulmonary embolism: preliminary results. Eur J Radiol 80(3):e505–e509
30. Apfaltrer P et al (2012) Prognostic value of perfusion defect volume at dual energy CTA in patients with pulmonary embolism: correlation with CTA obstruction scores, CT parameters of right ventricular dysfunction and adverse clinical outcome. Eur J Radiol 81(11):3592–3597
31. Bauer RW et al (2011) Dual energy CT pulmonary blood volume assessment in acute pulmonary embolism - correlation with D-dimer level, right heart strain and clinical outcome. Eur Radiol 21(9):1914–1921
32. Kang MJ et al (2010) Focal iodine defects on color-coded iodine perfusion maps of dual-energy pulmonary CT angiography images: a potential diagnostic pitfall. AJR Am J Roentgenol 195(5):W325–W330
33. Kim BH et al (2012) Analysis of perfusion defects by causes other than acute pulmonary thromboembolism on contrast-enhanced dual-energy CT in consecutive 537 patients. Eur J Radiol 81(4):e647–e652
34. Meinel FG et al (2013) Influence of vascular enhancement, age and gender on pulmonary perfused blood volume quantified by dual-energy-CTPA. Eur J Radiol 82(9):1565–1570
35. Copley SJ et al (2012) Effect of aging on lung structure in vivo: assessment with densitometric and fractal analysis of high-resolution computed tomography data. J Thorac Imaging 27(6): 366–371

36. Fuld MK et al (2013) Optimization of dual-energy xenon-computed tomography for quantitative assessment of regional pulmonary ventilation. Invest Radiol 48(9):629–637
37. Goo HW et al (2010) Xenon ventilation CT using dual-source and dual-energy technique in children with bronchiolitis obliterans: correlation of xenon and CT density values with pulmonary function test results. Pediatr Radiol 40(9):1490–1497
38. Park EA et al (2010) Chronic obstructive pulmonary disease: quantitative and visual ventilation pattern analysis at xenon ventilation CT performed by using a dual-energy technique. Radiology 256(3):985–997
39. Zhang LJ, Zhou CS, Lu GM (2012) Dual energy computed tomography demonstrated lung ventilation/perfusion mismatch in a 19-year-old patient with pulmonary embolism. Circulation 126(20):2441–2443
40. Zhang LJ et al (2013) Dual-energy CT lung ventilation/perfusion imaging for diagnosing pulmonary embolism. Eur Radiol 23(10):2666–2675
41. Meinel FG et al (2012) Metal artifact reduction by dual-energy computed tomography using energetic extrapolation: a systematically optimized protocol. Invest Radiol 47(7):406–414
42. Delesalle MA et al (2013) Spectral optimization of chest CT angiography with reduced iodine load: experience in 80 patients evaluated with dual-source, dual-energy CT. Radiology 267(1):256–266
43. Cheng J et al (2013) Optimal monochromatic energy levels in spectral CT pulmonary angiography for the evaluation of pulmonary embolism. PLoS One 8(5), e63140
44. Schenzle JC et al (2010) Dual energy CT of the chest: how about the dose? Invest Radiol 45(6):347–353
45. Henzler T et al (2012) Dual-energy CT: radiation dose aspects. AJR Am J Roentgenol 199 (5 Suppl):S16–S25
46. Meinel FG et al (2014) Radiation risks from cardiovascular imaging tests. Circulation 130(5):442–445
47. Keylock JB, Galvin JR, Franks TJ (2009) Sclerosing hemangioma of the lung. Arch Pathol Lab Med 133(5):820–825

Dual Energy CT in Liver Tumors

5

Carlo N. De Cecco, Julian L. Wichmann,
Giuseppe Muscogiuri, Andrew Hardie, and Andrea Laghi

5.1 Introduction

Dual energy computed tomography (DECT) is an innovative imaging technique, whose basic principle is the application of two separate low- and high-energy tube voltages during the CT acquisition enabling the transition from density-based imaging to spectral imaging.

DECT applications in liver imaging are based on two distinct capabilities: (1) material differentiation and (2) material identification and quantification. The possibility to obtain different material-specific (iodine mapping and virtual unenhanced

C.N. De Cecco, MD, PhD (✉) • G. Muscogiuri, MD
Department of Radiology and Radiological Science, Medical University of South Carolina, 25 Courtenay Drive, Charleston, SC 29425, USA

Department of Radiological Sciences, Oncology and Pathology, University of Rome "Sapienza", Rome, Italy
e-mail: dececco@musc.edu; muscogiu@musc.edu

J.L. Wichmann, MD
Department of Radiology and Radiological Science, Medical University of South Carolina, 25 Courtenay Drive, Charleston, SC 29425, USA

Department of Diagnostic and Interventional Radiology, University Hospital Frankfurt, Frankfurt, Germany
e-mail: wichmann@musc.edu

A. Hardie, MD
Department of Radiology and Radiological Science, Medical University of South Carolina, 25 Courtenay Drive, Charleston, SC 29425, USA
e-mail: hardie@musc.edu

A. Laghi, MD
Department of Radiological Sciences, Oncology and Pathology, University of Rome "Sapienza", Rome, Italy
e-mail: andrea.laghi@uniroma1.it

© Springer International Publishing Switzerland 2015
C.N. De Cecco et al. (eds.), *Dual Energy CT in Oncology*,
DOI 10.1007/978-3-319-19563-6_5

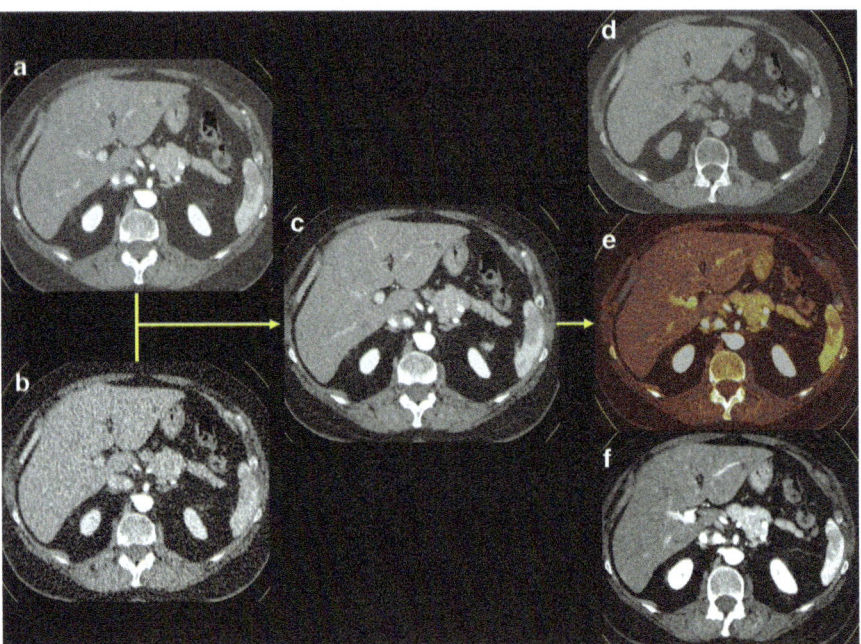

Fig. 5.1 DECT post-processing workflow. (**a**) 100 kVp dataset, (**b**) Sn150 kVp dataset, (**c**) 120 kV mixed image, (**d**) virtual unenhanced image, (**e**) color-coded iodine map, (**f**) virtual monoenergetic image (50 keV)

(VU) images) or energy-specific (virtual monoenergetic images) datasets during a single scan may provide several advantages in oncological imaging [1] (Fig. 5.1).

The calculation of VU images may replace the acquisition of pre-contrast images, therefore substantially lowering the radiation burden especially in younger patients who are more at risk for radiation-induced consequences or patients who undergo repeated follow-up CT examinations. Iodine maps can be useful to improve visualization and detection of contrast uptake, potentially increasing the diagnostic confidence for assessment of metastatic lesion contrast enhancement or conversely ruling out the presence of any contrast enhancement in small benign cystic lesions. Virtual monoenergetic images at low energy levels are beneficial in increasing image contrast, thus potentially improving the visualization and assessment of both hypovascular and hypervascular liver lesions. Due to increased image contrast, virtual monoenergetic imaging may also allow for a reduction of contrast material administered. These capabilities may have beneficial effects on the detection of cancer-related comorbidities and the evaluation of treatment response (Table. 5.1) [2]. All these applications, if routinely applied, could improve the safety of CT examinations by reducing the radiation dose and contrast medium amount administered, while at the same time enhancing the detection and characterization of liver lesions.

Table 5.1 Advantages of DECT datasets in liver imaging

DECT of liver tumors	
Dataset	Advantages
Virtual unenhanced	Replacement of conventional unenhanced acquisition
	Radiation dose reduction
Iodine mapping	Intralesional iodine detection
	Iodine uptake quantification
	Response to therapy assessment
Virtual monoenergetic	Liver lesion detection
	Liver lesion conspicuity
	Contrast material reduction

5.2   Material-Specific Applications

5.2.1   Virtual Unenhanced Images

Material-specific images may be used for determining the presence and quantity of materials with unique absorption characteristics, including chemical elements such as iodine, iron, calcium, and gadolinium, or compound materials such as fat, uric acid, or blood.

In particular, detection and computed removal of iodine enables the calculation of VU images, which may obviate the need of routine conventional unenhanced (CU) scans (Fig. 5.2). This may be of special relevance in follow-up liver CT, which is commonly performed using biphasic or triphasic scan protocols which result in a relatively high radiation dose. VU images may allow for a reduction of approximately 30 % in clinical practice [3–6].

First- and second-generation dual-source DECT abdominal VU datasets, despite mostly excellent image quality, were not ready to replace CU images in clinical practice due to limitations that could impair diagnostic accuracy such as inhomogeneous iodine subtraction and reduction in the attenuation of calcifications and metallic clips [3–6]. In particular, inhomogeneous iodine subtraction has been reported in the presence of high iodine concentration, e.g., in small peripheral liver vessels. A lack of contrast subtraction on VU images has also been observed in the case of liver metastasis as a ring artifact around the lesion. Furthermore, erroneous calcium subtraction was shown and could interfere with characterization of calcified liver lesions. While these artifacts do not affect the image quality, they could be the source of pitfalls in certain clinical cases.

Recently, third-generation dual-source CT has become commercially available that provides several technological innovations which may be beneficial in DECT. A preliminary report on VU images reconstructed with this scanner demonstrated good quality of VU images and, unlike second generation, a complete subtraction of liver iodine has been reported [7] (Fig. 5.3). However, the issue of erroneous

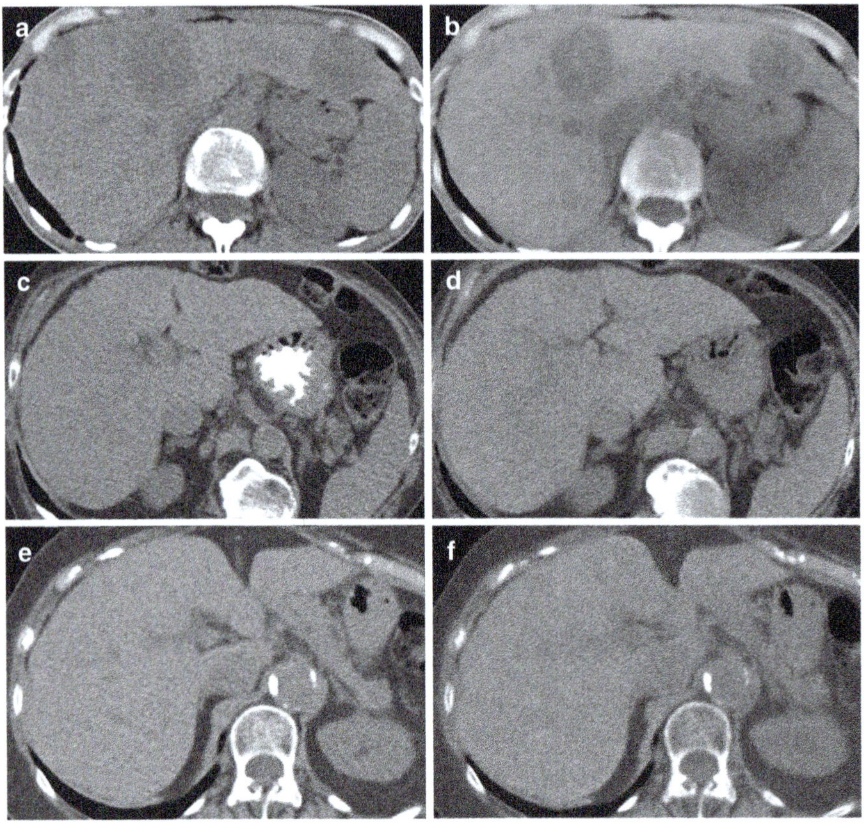

Fig. 5.2 Comparison of virtual unenhanced images obtained with dual-source dual-energy scanners from different generations. (**a, c, e**) Conventional unenhanced datasets obtained with first, second, and third generation dual-source dual-energy CT, respectively; (**b, d, f**) corresponding virtual unenhanced images reconstructed from the venous phase. A significant improvement in image quality and iodine subtraction from the liver parenchyma is evident in each generation compared to the last

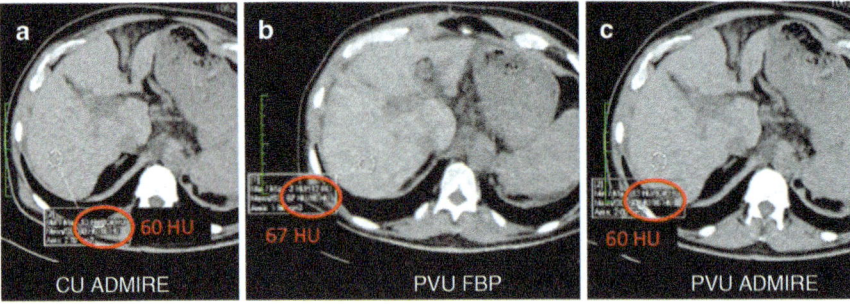

Fig. 5.3 Third-generation conventional (**a**) and virtual unenhanced (**b, c**) datasets from the venous phase reconstructed with filtered back projection (FBP) and advanced modeled iterative reconstruction algorithm (ADMIRE, strength 3). Virtual unenhanced datasets show similar liver attenuation values as conventional unenhanced images, demonstrating a complete subtraction of contrast signal from the liver parenchyma. ADMIRE significantly improved overall image quality

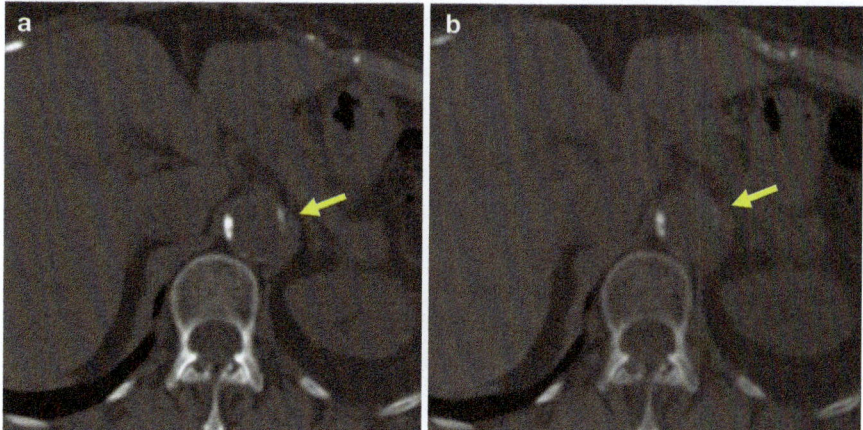

Fig. 5.4 Third-generation conventional unenhanced image (**a**) and virtual unenhanced image from the arterial phase (**b**). A reduction in the attenuation of aortic calcifications (*arrow*) can be observed in the virtual unenhanced dataset

subtraction of calcified aortic lesions (Fig. 5.4) and metallic clips persists, as it is intrinsic to the technique; thus, radiologists should be aware of these limitations when incorporating VU datasets into their DECT protocols.

Future improvements in DECT post-processing may alleviate these issues to transform VU image reconstruction into a routine technique in DECT to reduce radiation exposure.

5.2.2 Iodine Mapping

DECT-derived maps of iodine distribution in the liver parenchyma can be used to identify iodine uptake in tumors and can act as a surrogate for lesion vascularization. In fact, DECT can provide a direct and accurate quantification of the iodine uptake in milligrams per milliliters (mg/ml) (Fig. 5.5). Besides its diagnostic value for lesion characterization (i.e., differential diagnosis of a hepatic lesion too small to differentiate between a tiny cyst and a solid metastasis) (Fig. 5.6), DECT iodine maps may also be beneficial for the assessment of lesion response after therapy.

Recently, the assessment of lesion-specific iodine concentration has been used to differentiate hepatic hemangiomas from hepatocellular carcinoma (HCC) [8]. Atypical hemangiomas, which are frequently observed in patients with liver cirrhosis, represent an imaging challenge when attempting to differentiate them from HCC [9]. The capability to employ quantification of iodine concentration to differentiate these two entities may render DECT an important tool in the surveillance of cirrhotic liver parenchyma. Furthermore, in patients with colorectal carcinoma, the early detection of liver metastasis may positively impact treatment options and outcome. In the presence of small liver nodules in these patients, the reliable differentiation of small benign cysts from metastasis may not be feasible with CT in cases. The accurate detection and assessment of iodine in the lesion may thus improve the diagnostic confidence for lesion characterization [1].

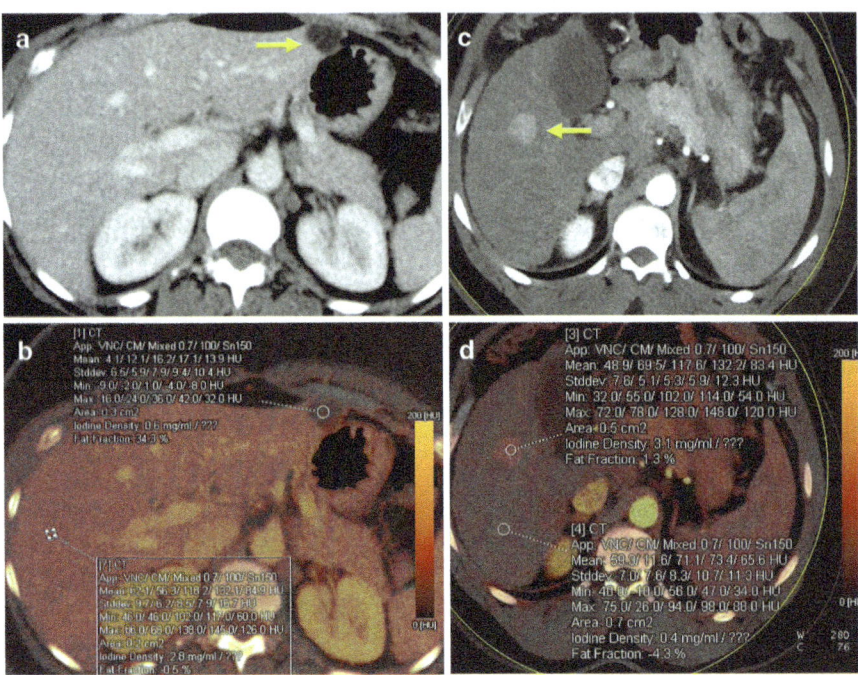

Fig. 5.5 DECT-derived maps of iodine distribution in the liver parenchyma can be used to identify and quantify iodine uptake of liver lesions. (**a, b**) Benign cystic lesion (*arrow*) showing no contrast enhancement (iodine density: 0.6 mg/ml) in comparison with the liver parenchyma in the venous phase (iodine density: 2.8 mg/ml). (**c, d**) HCC nodule with significant iodine uptake (iodine density: 3.1 mg/ml) during the arterial phase in comparison with the surrounding liver parenchyma (iodine density: 0.4 mg/ml). *HCC* hepatocarcinoma

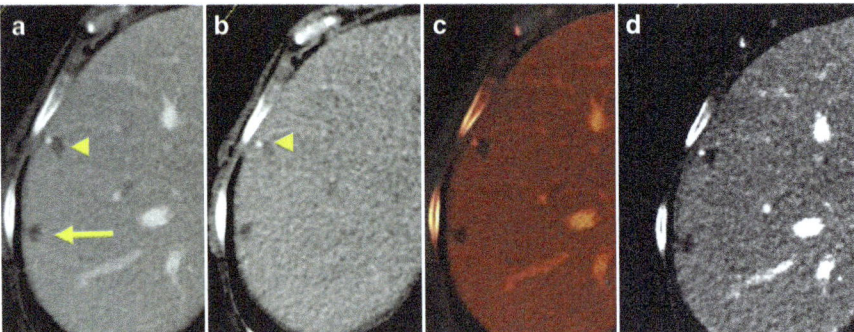

Fig. 5.6 The combination of virtual unenhanced images and iodine maps can be used to improve diagnostic confidence in liver lesion characterization. In patients with colorectal cancer, the discrimination of small liver cysts from metastatic disease can represent a diagnostic dilemma (**a**, *arrow* and *arrowhead*). Virtual unenhanced images (**b**) demonstrate the presence of a small lesion with calcification (*arrowhead*). Iodine-based maps (**c, d**) show the absence of any intralesional contrast uptake, suggesting a diagnosis of benign liver cysts

5.3   Energy-Specific Applications

5.3.1   Low kVp Images

A general advantage of DECT in liver imaging is the possibility to simultaneously obtain two different image datasets at low (80–100 kVp) and high (140–150 kVp) tube voltages and therefore energy spectra.

Since in low kV datasets are acquired with energy levels closer to the k-edge of iodine, a mean significant increase in attenuation can be observed, in particular in contrast-enhanced structures. This represents a well-known advantage in vascular studies in which a significant increase in signal-to-noise ratio (SNR) and contrast-to-noise ratio (CNR) can be achieved, with better visualization of contrast-enhanced vessels, accompanied by a distinct reduction in radiation dose in SE acquisition. This approach can also be applied to the detection of hypervascular liver lesions. For the evaluation of late arterial phase 80-kVp datasets in comparison to standard 120-kVp images, several studies demonstrated a significant improvement in HCC detection and lesion conspicuity (Fig. 5.7). Apparently, the associated increase in image noise does not impair detection of small hepatic lesions [10, 11]. However, Park et al. did not observe an improvement in HCC detection with 80-kVp images despite significantly higher CNR [12]. Since the increased attenuation of iodine in low-kVp images comes at the cost of increased image noise, overall image quality and CNR may be lower especially in obese patients. Nevertheless, the recently introduced third-generation DSCT system provides higher tube currents in low-kVp imaging which may overcome this limitation.

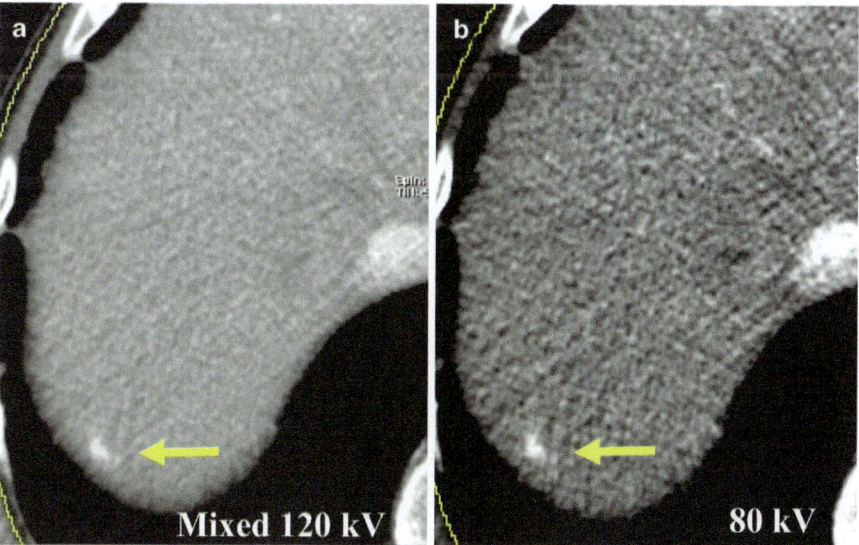

Fig. 5.7 Small hypervascular liver lesion best detected on an 80 kV dataset (**b**) in comparison to a mixed 120 kV image (**a**)

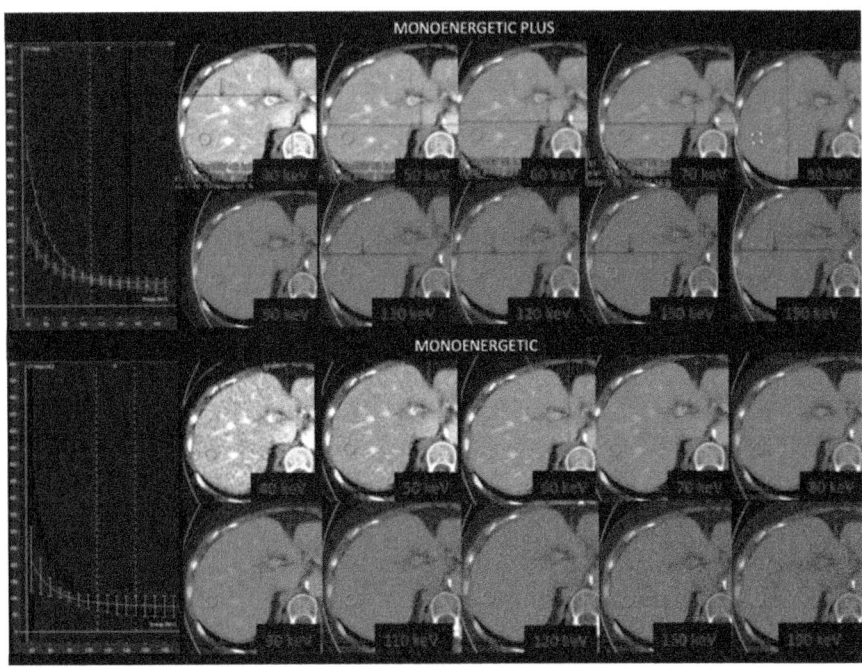

Fig. 5.8 Virtual monoenergetic datasets. Low energy levels (40–70 keV) are beneficial in increasing contrast attenuation, potentially improving the visualization and assessment of both hypovascular and hypervascular liver lesions. Mono + significantly improves the image quality of monoenergetic datasets at low keV levels by substantially reducing the image noise

Similar to the results reported for imaging of hypervascular liver lesions, promising results have also been reported in a small cohort of patients affected by hypovascular hepatic metastases, in whom a significant increase in CNR between metastatic lesions and normal liver parenchyma was observed during portal venous phase acquisition at 80 kVp [13]. However, the potential improvement in attenuation and thus visualization of hypovascular liver lesions appears limited compared to imaging of hypervascular liver lesions on arterial-phase scans, in whom this approach should be preferably used.

5.3.2   Virtual Monoenergetic Images

Dedicated post-processing of DECT datasets also provides the possibility to reconstruct virtual monoenergetic images (also referred in literature as virtual monochromatic) at selected hypothetical x-ray photon energy levels from a standard polychromatic examination (Fig. 5.8). This approach can be effective to substantially improve CNR and thus lesion detectability but can also be used in the setting of tissue characterization by analyzing attenuation curves of different materials at distinct energy levels.

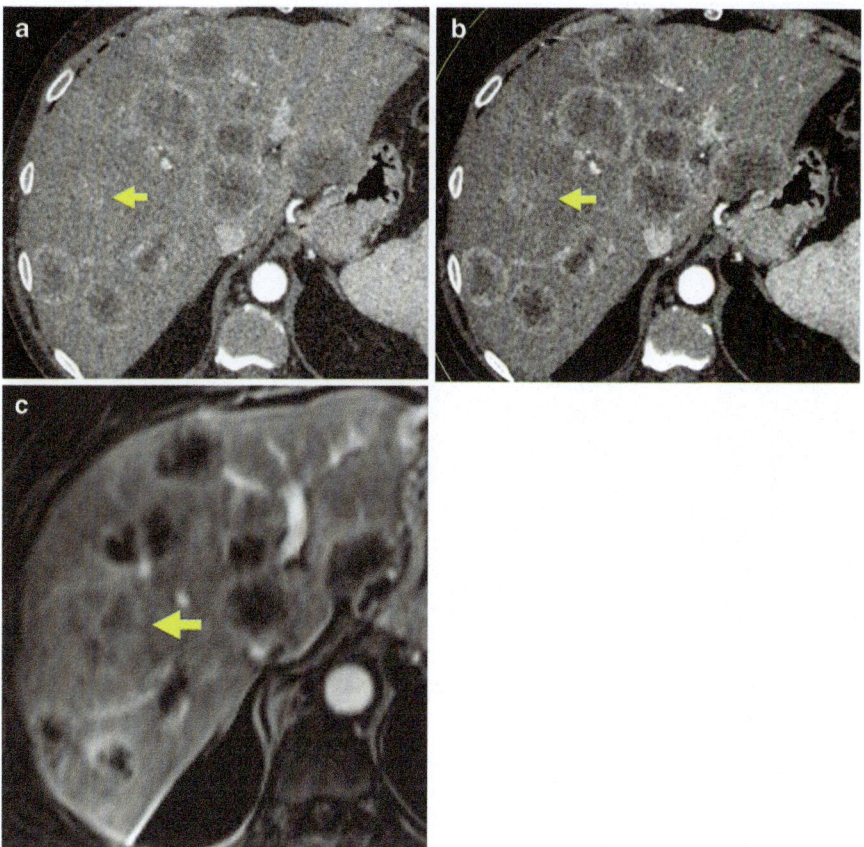

Fig. 5.9 Patient with lung cancer and multiple liver metastases with central necrosis. In the mono-chromatic dataset at 50 keV (**b**), lesion conspicuity is significantly enhanced compared to mixed 120 kV image (**a**), improving the visualization of liver lesions and the detection of nodules (*arrow*) usually assessable only with magnetic resonance (**c**)

Several prior studies investigated the application of this technique in clinical practice, demonstrating that with the traditional monoenergetic algorithm the best CNR in contrast-enhanced DECT is usually achieved at 70–75 keV. Further lowering of the energy level usually results in excessive image noise which diminishes the potential benefits of increased iodine attenuation [14, 15].

Recently, a novel monoenergetic algorithm (Mono+) has been released with the goal to improve the image quality of monoenergetic datasets at low keV levels (40 keV) by substantially reducing the image noise using an advanced image-based algorithm [16]. Promising initial results from clinical studies have been reported and their potential to significantly improve the visualization of hypervascular and hypovascular liver lesions has been demonstrated [17, 18] (Fig. 5.9).

Preliminary evidence suggests that the use of reconstructed virtual monoenergetic images at lower energy levels (40–70 keV) can significantly improve the conspicuity

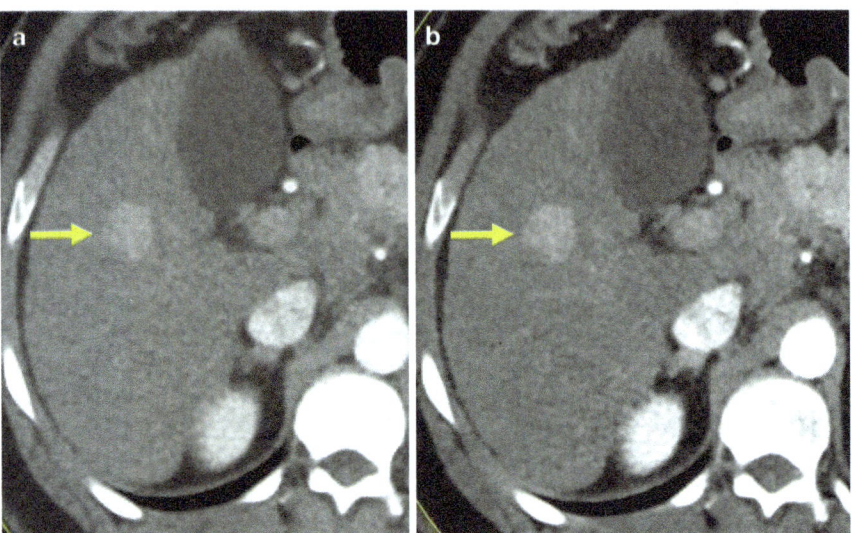

Fig. 5.10 Virtual monoenergetic imaging at a low energy level (50 keV) (**b**) significantly improves the conspicuity and detection of hypervascular liver lesion (*arrow*) in comparison with mixed 120 kV image (**a**). *HCC* hepatocarcinoma

and detection rate of small hypervascular liver lesions [19] (Fig. 5.10). Similarly, higher CNR between hypovascular liver metastases and adjacent parenchyma was demonstrated for low keV reconstructions of portal-venous-phase images compared to standard DECT images [20]. A similarly improved lesion conspicuity and increased rate of visible hyperenhancing lesions were noted at lower keV levels in a multireader pilot study in a population of patients with liver cirrhosis undergoing surveillance DECT for early detection of hepatocellular carcinoma [21].

Finally, low-keV monoenergetic images may also allow for a reduction of the amount of contrast material administered while maintaining an adequate parenchymal attenuation and image quality. This approach could be useful to improve safety and examination protocols in patients with impaired renal function.

5.4   Evaluation of Response to Therapy

New drugs targeted toward cellular neoangiogenesis and growth molecular mechanisms have substantially changed the requirements for imaging modalities of tumor response. The traditional criteria used to assess response to therapy, mainly based on lesion number and size (e.g., RECIST) [22], are insufficient to provide reliable assessment of tumor response to target drugs.

For example, gastrointestinal stromal tumors (GIST) may not show size reduction following therapy with imatinib, but merely a dramatic change in density. For this reason, new criteria based on CT attenuation changes have been proposed [23]. However, the presence of therapy-related intra-tumoral hemorrhage can also affect

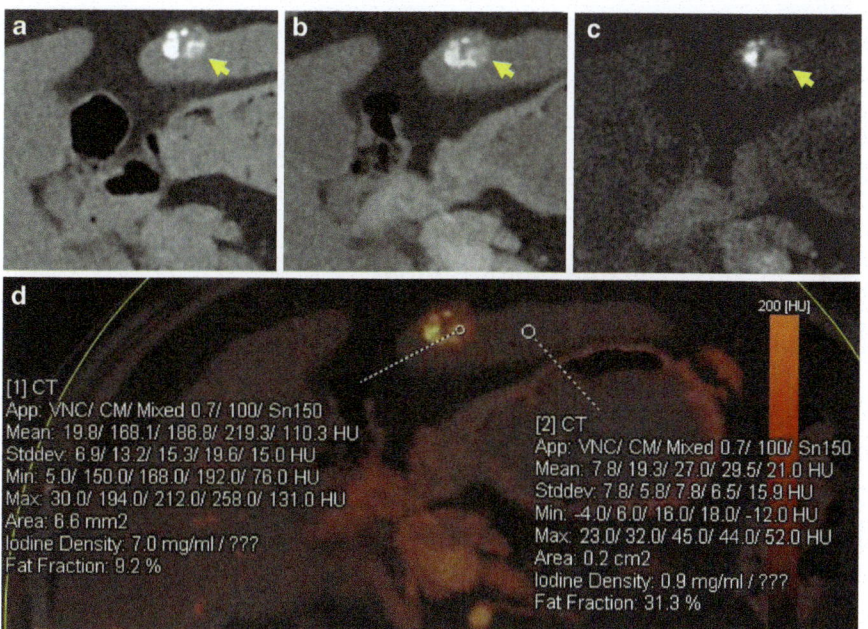

Fig. 5.11 Tumor recurrence after TACE in HCC. Conventional unenhanced dataset (**a**) shows the presence of residual hyperdense material in the treated lesion (*arrow*), limiting the evaluation of post-contrast enhancement due to tumor recurrence (**b**, *arrow*). Iodine map helps in detecting viable tumor tissue (**c**, *arrow*); iodine uptake is confirmed by quantitative analysis of the nodule (**d**, iodine density 7.0 mg/ml). *TACE* transarterial chemoembolization, *HCC* hepatocarcinoma

the assessment of post-contrast tumoral density. In a recent study [24], the possibilty to use DECT VU images as baseline reference and iodine-based datasets to accurately assess intratumoral amount of iodinated contrast medium has been considered to establish surrogate parameters of lesion perfusion and vascularization.

In addition, the capability to accurately detect parenchymal iodine distribution within an iodine-based image could permit better quantification of subtle tumor vascularization and response to antiangiogenic therapy, radiofrequency ablation, or selective internal radiation therapy (Fig. 5.11).

The application of iodine maps for the evaluation of HCC angiogenesis instead of perfusion CT has also been recently investigated in animal studies [25]. Preliminary results demonstrated a significant correlation between attenuation values of viable tumor tissue measured in iodine maps and the corresponding perfusion CT values, indicating the potential of DECT for evaluation of tumor response to therapy instead of perfusion CT would allow for significant total radiation exposure savings.

Iodine maps and VU images may also possess diagnostic value in the assessment of HCC response to radiofrequency ablation [26] or transarterial chemoembolization [27]. Iodine maps can improve conspicuity of the ablation zone especially because of its excellent internal homogeneity and sharp ablative margins. Higher lesion-to-liver CNR on iodine maps can also be helpful for detecting residual viable tumor tissue.

Furthermore, the accurate detection and quantification of iodine concentration on iodine-mapping images can be used as a more reliable and reproducible bio-marker of tumor vascularity and may predict the likelihood of tumor response to antiangiogenic therapy [28–30].

5.5   Cancer-Related Comorbidities

In oncologic patients, several complications directly caused by cancer treatment or tumor manifestation itself can occur at any time. DECT can also play a crucial role in the detection of early cancer-related comorbidities. For example, iodine mapping or virtual monoenergetic images can be used in patients with liver tumors to detect vascular invasion and thrombosis associated with HCC or in case of suspected pulmonary thromboembolism [1]. In particular, the improvement in CNR obtained by evaluating low-keV monoenergetic datasets could significantly improve the detection of portal venous thrombosis caused by vascular invasion from HCC. Similarly, iodine detection and quantification has demonstrated advantages in the identification of tumoral thrombus in patients with HCC and vena cava invasion, as this technique is particularly helpful in the differentiation of malignant from benign thrombosis [31].

5.6   Radiation Dose Considerations

Concerns about possible additional radiation dose with DE acquisition have been stated since two separate datasets are obtained at different tube voltages. However, different technical realizations of DECT have also varying impact on radiation exposure.

In fast kilovoltage-switching dual-energy CT, tube current modulation and fil-tration of the two x-ray energies cannot be independently performed, therefore slightly increasing the radiation dose by approximately 15 % in comparison with SE acquisition [32].

Phantom and patient studies performed with first- and second-generation DSCT systems with automated attenuation-based dose modulation concluded that DE acquisition delivers the same amount of radiation in comparison with traditional 120 kV SE acquisition [33, 34] or even less with reduced tube current [35, 36]. Third-generation DSCT has also been confirmed to be dose-neutral in comparison with SE acquisition [7]. Thus, DE acquisition can be routinely used on that system, in particular when additional diagnostic information with a potential impact on patient management can be expected from spectral acquisition and analysis.

Conclusion
In conclusion, DECT provides several beneficial applications in liver imaging. The possibility to obtain different material-specific and energy-specific datasets during a single scan can improve detection and characterization of liver lesions.

This approach can also be auxiliary in the prediction and evaluation of tumor response to therapy and in the detection of cancer-related comorbidities and complications.

References

1. De Cecco CN, Darnell A, Rengo M, Muscogiuri G, Bellini D, Ayuso C, Laghi A (2012) Dual-energy CT: oncologic applications. AJR Am J Roentgenol 199(5 Suppl):S98–S105
2. Marin D, Boll DT, Mileto A, Nelson RC (2014) State of the art: dual-energy CT of the abdomen. Radiology 271(2):327–342
3. De Cecco CN, Buffa V, Fedeli S, Luzietti M, Vallone A, Ruopoli R, Miele V et al (2010) Dual energy CT (DECT) of the liver: conventional virtual unenhanced images. Eur Radiol 20:2870–2875
4. Zhang LJ, Peng J, Wu SY, Wang ZJ, Wu XS, Zhou CS, Ji XM, Lu GM (2010) Liver virtual non-enhanced CT with dual-source, dual-energy CT: a preliminary study. Eur Radiol 20:2257–2264
5. De Cecco CN, Buffa V, Fedeli S, Vallone A, Ruopoli R, Luzietti M, Miele V et al (2010) Preliminary experience with dual energy CT (DECT) of the abdomen: real versus virtual non-enhanced images of the liver. Radiol Med 115:1258–1266
6. De Cecco CN, Darnell A, Macías N, Ayuso JR, Rodríguez S, Rimola J, Pagés M, García-Criado A, Rengo M, Laghi A, Ayuso C (2013) Virtual unenhanced images of the abdomen with second-generation dual-source dual-energy computed tomography: image quality and liver lesion detection. Invest Radiol 48(1):1–9
7. De Cecco CN, Spearman J, Schoepf UJ, Canstein C, Meinel FG, Hardie A (2014) Virtual unenhanced images of the abdomen with 3rd generation dual-source dual-energy CT and 3rd generation iterative reconstruction: image quality, attenuation and radiation dose. RSNA 2014, Chicago
8. Lv P, Lin XZ, Li J, Li W, Chen K (2011) Differentiation of small hepatic hemangioma from small hepatocellular carcinoma: recently introduced spectral CT method. Radiology 259(3):720–729
9. Kim T, Federle MP, Baron RL, Peterson MS, Kawamori Y (2001) Discrimination of small hepatic hemangiomas from hypervascular malignant tumors smaller than 3 cm with three-phase helical CT. Radiology 219(3):699–706
10. Marin D, Nelson RC, Samei E et al (2009) Hypervascular liver tumors: low tube voltage, high tube current multidetector CT during late hepatic arterial phase for detection – initial clinical experience. Radiology 251:771–779
11. Altenbernd J, Heusner TA, Ringelstein A, Ladd SC, Forsting M, Antoch G (2011) Dual-energy-CT of hypervascular liver lesions in patients with HCC: investigation of image quality and sensitivity. Eur Radiol 21:738–743
12. Park JK, Kim SH, Park HS, Kim GH, Lee JY et al (2011) Added value of 80 kVp images to averaged 120 kVp images in the detection of hepatocellular carcinoma in liver transplantation candidates using dual-source dual-energy MDCT: results of JAFROC analysis. Eur J Radiol 80:e76–e85
13. Robinson E, Babb J, Chandarana H, Macari M (2010) Dual source dual energy MDCT comparison of 80 kVp and weighted average 120 kVp data for conspicuity of hypo-vascular liver metastases. Invest Radiol 45:413–418
14. Morgan DE (2014) Dual-energy CT, of the abdomen. Abdom Imaging 39(1):108–134
15. Yu L, Leng S, McCollough CH (2012) Dual-energy CT-based monochromatic imaging. AJR Am J Roentgenol 199(5 Suppl):S9–S15
16. Grant KL, Flohr TG, Krauss B, Sedlmair M, Thomas C, Schmidt B (2014) Assessment of an advanced image-based technique to calculate virtual monoenergetic computed tomographic images from a dual-energy examination to improve contrast-to-noise ratio in examinations using iodinated contrast media. Invest Radiol 49(9):586–592

17. De Cecco CN, Spearman J, Schoepf UJ, Canstein C, Meinel FG, Hardie A (2014) Value of an advanced image-based technique to calculate virtual monoenergetic CT images using third-generation dual-energy dual-source CT to improve contrast-to-noise ratio in liver examinations. RSNA 2014, Chicago
18. Albrecht MH, Scholtz JE, Kraft J, Bauer RW, Kaup M, Dewes P, Bucher AM, Burck I, Wagenblast J, Lehnert T, Kerl JM, Vogl TJ, Wichmann JL (2015) Assessment of an advanced monoenergetic reconstruction technique in dual-energy computed tomography of head and neck cancer. Eur Radiol 2015 Feb 14. [Epub ahead of print]
19. Lv P, Lin XZ, Chen K, Gao J (2012) Spectral CT in patients with small HCC: investigation of image quality and diagnostic accuracy. Eur Radiol 22(10):2117–2124
20. Yamada Y, Jinzaki M, Tanami Y, Abe T, Kuribayashi S (2012) Virtual monochromatic spectral imaging for the evaluation of hypovascular hepatic metastases: the optimal monochromatic level with fast kilovoltage switching dual-energy computed tomography. Invest Radiol 47: 292–298
21. Thomas JV, Alexander L, Bolus D, Morgan DE (2011) Evaluation of lesion conspicuity of hepatocellular carcinomas (HCC) in cirrhotics using dual energy spectral MDCT. ARRS Annual Meeting, Chicago
22. Choi H, Charnsangavej C, de Castro Faria S et al (2004) CT evaluation of the response of gastrointestinal stromal tumors after imatinib mesylate treatment: a quantitative analysis correlated with FDG PET finding. Am J Roentgenol 183:1619–1628
23. Apfaltrer P, Meyer M, Meier C, Henzler T, Barraza JM, Dinter DJ et al (2012) Contrast-enhanced dual-energy CT of gastrointestinal stromal tumors. Is iodine-related attenuation a potential indicator of tumor response. Invest Radiol 47:65–70
24. Schlemmer M, Sourbron SP, Schinwald N et al (2011) Perfusion patterns of metastatic gastro-intestinal stromal tumor lesion under specific molecular therapy. Eur J Radiol 77:312–318
25. Zhanga LJ, Wub S, Wanga M, Lua L, Chena B, Jin L et al (2012) Quantitative dual energy CT measurements in rabbit VX2 liver tumors: comparison to perfusion CT measurements and histopathological findings. Eur J Radiol 81:1766–1775
26. Lee SH, Lee JM, Kim KW et al (2011) Dual-energy computed tomography to assess tumor response to hepatic radiofrequency ablation: potential diagnostic values of virtual noncontrast images and iodine maps. Invest Radiol 46:77–84
27. Lee JA, Jeong WK, Kim Y et al (2013) Dual-energy CT to detect recurrent HCC after TACE: initial experience of color-coded iodine CT imaging. Eur J Radiol 82:569–576
28. Chen B, Marin D, Richard S, Husarik D, Nelson R, Samei E (2013) Precision of iodine quantification in hepatic CT: effects of iterative reconstruction with various imaging parameters. AJR Am J Roentgenol 200(5):W475–W482
29. Dai X, Schlemmer HP, Schmidt B et al (2013) Quantitative therapy response assessment by volumetric iodine-uptake measurement: initial experience in patients with advanced hepatocellular carcinoma treated with sorafenib. Eur J Radiol 82(2):327–334
30. Komatsu S, Fukumoto T, Demizu Y et al (2011) Clinical results and risk factors of proton and carbon ion therapy for hepatocellular carcinoma. Cancer 117(21):4890–4904
31. Qian LJ, Zhu J, Zhuang ZG et al (2012) Differentiation of neoplastic from bland macroscopic portal vein thrombi using dual-energy spectral CT imaging: a pilot study. Eur Radiol 22: 2178–2185
32. Zou Y, Silver MD (2009) Analysis of fast kV-switching in dual energy CT using a pre-reconstruction decomposition technique. In: Hsieh J, Samei E, eds. Proceedings of SPIE: medical imaging 2008—physics of medical imaging, vol 6913. SPIE–The International Society for Optic Engineering, Bellingham, p 691313
33. Christner JA, Kofler JM, McCollough CH (2010) Estimating effective dose for CT using dose–length product compared with using organ doses: consequences of adopting international commission on radiological protection publication 103 or dual-energy scanning. Am J Roentgenol 194:881–889

34. Schenzle JC, Sommer WH, Neumaier K, Michalski G, Lechel U et al (2010) Dual energy CT of the chest How about the dose? Invest Radiol 45:347–353
35. De Zordo T, von Lutterotti K, Dejaco C, Soegner PF, Frank R et al (2012) Comparison of image quality and radiation dose of different pulmonary CTA protocols on a 128-slice CT: high-pitch dual source CT, dual energy CT and conventional spiral CT. Eur Radiol 22:279–286
36. Bauer RW, Kramer S, Renker M, Schell B, Larson MC et al (2011) Dose and image quality at CT pulmonary angiography – comparison of first and second generation dual-energy CT and 64-slice CT. Eur Radiol 21:2139–2147

Dual Energy CT in Pancreatic Tumors

6

Desiree E. Morgan

6.1   Introduction

Since 2010, when Macari et al. [1] first published a report on initial observations using dual energy CT in patients with pancreas adenocarcinoma, the utility of this new technology for evaluation of pancreatic neoplasms has been explored not only for pancreatic adenocarcinoma, but also for pancreatic neuroendocrine neoplasms and cystic pancreatic lesions. This chapter will provide an update of the application of dual energy acquisition, image generation, and postprocessing to enhance visualization and characterization of focal pancreatic tumors. Dynamic imaging with dual energy CT provides two advantageous categories of images that are not available with standard single energy MDCT: Low kVp images and/or simulated monoenergetic images, and material specific images (Fig. 6.1). Simulated monoenergetic and low kVp imaging are used to improve lesion contrast and conspicuity. Material density imaging is important not only for identification of focal lesions within the pancreas and other organs, but also potentially for determining the presence and quantity of tissue iodine before and during neoadjuvant or adjuvant therapy. In addition, materials other than iodine: Elements such as iron, calcium, and gadolinium; or materials such as fat, uric acid, blood, or even mucin can be evaluated. The presentation of the dual energy information varies among manufacturers and there is an opportunity for practitioners to optimize postprocessing to meet the needs of their practices (Fig. 6.2).

D.E. Morgan, MD
Department of Radiology, University of Alabama,
JT N452 619 19th Street South, Birmingham, AL 35249-6830, USA
e-mail: dmorgan@uabmc.edu

© Springer International Publishing Switzerland 2015
C.N. De Cecco et al. (eds.), *Dual Energy CT in Oncology*,
DOI 10.1007/978-3-319-19563-6_6

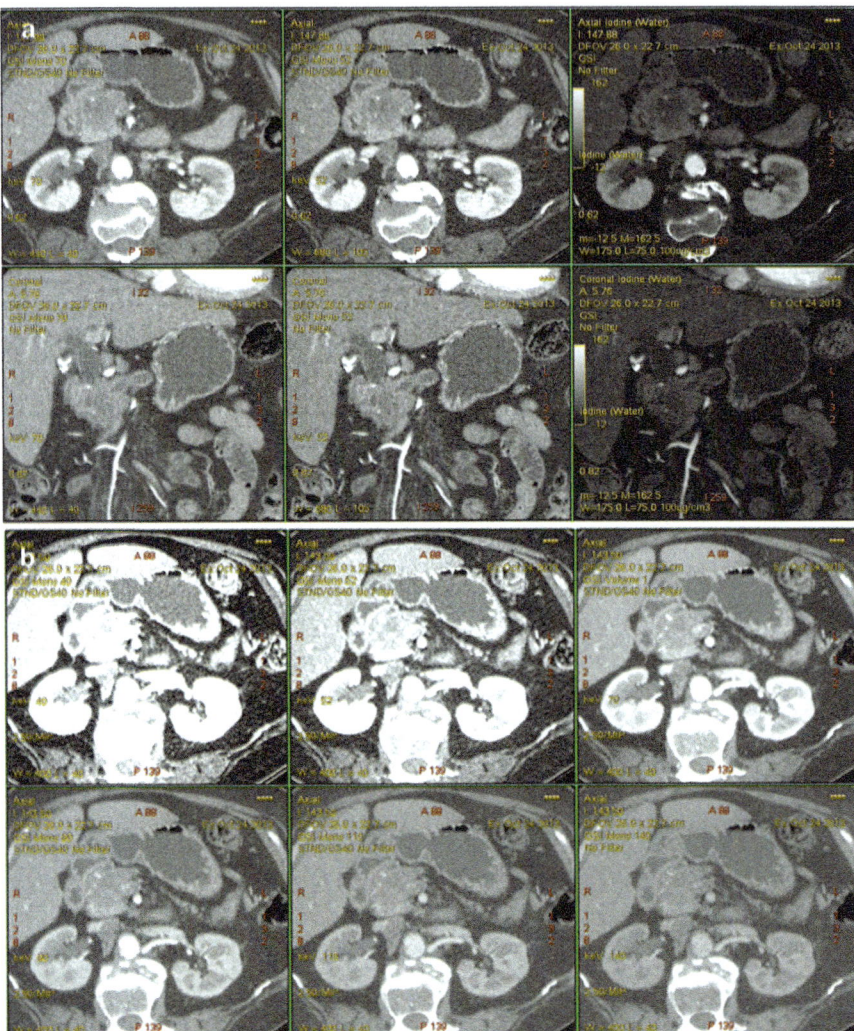

Fig. 6.1 A 66-year-old woman with pancreatic ductal adenocarcinoma. (**a**) DECT pancreatic parenchymal phase GSI server standard pancreatic carcinoma postprocessing "collage" with 70 keV (*left column*), 52 keV (*middle column*), iodine MD (*right column*), axial (*top*), and coronal (*bottom*) images demonstrate a large hypovascular mass in the anterior pancreatic head, encasing the gastroduodenal artery and abutting the unopacified SMV. The entrance of the obstructed pancreatic and bile ducts into the mass is best depicted on the coronal images. The margins appear sharper on the low energy and iodine images even though these are source 0.625 mm images. The images can be made to any desired thickness, and other image variables such as viewing keV, FOV, material decomposition basis pair, imaging plane, window, and level can be instantaneously adjusted. (**b**) GSI server collage demonstrating alteration in appearance of simulated monoenergetic images as the energy increases from 40 (*top left* to 140 (*bottom right*) keV. The window and level have been kept constant at 400/40 in order to show that the increased contrast/brightness is solely due to the change in viewing energy. Note that as the energy decreases, the amount of image noise increases. Our previous research has found that optimum pancreatic adenocarcinoma simulated monoenergetic viewing is in the low 50 keV range. (**c**) Same patient approximately 13 weeks later during neoadjuvant therapy with FOLFIRINOX. A metallic stent has been placed into the bile duct, and the tumor appears slightly smaller but continues to encase/abut the SMV. This patient was eventually resected with R0 margins

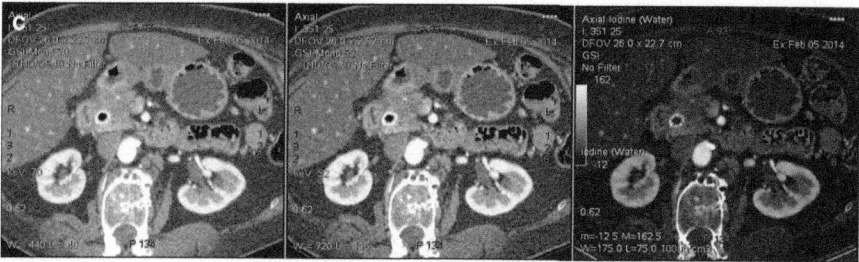

Fig. 6.1 (continued)

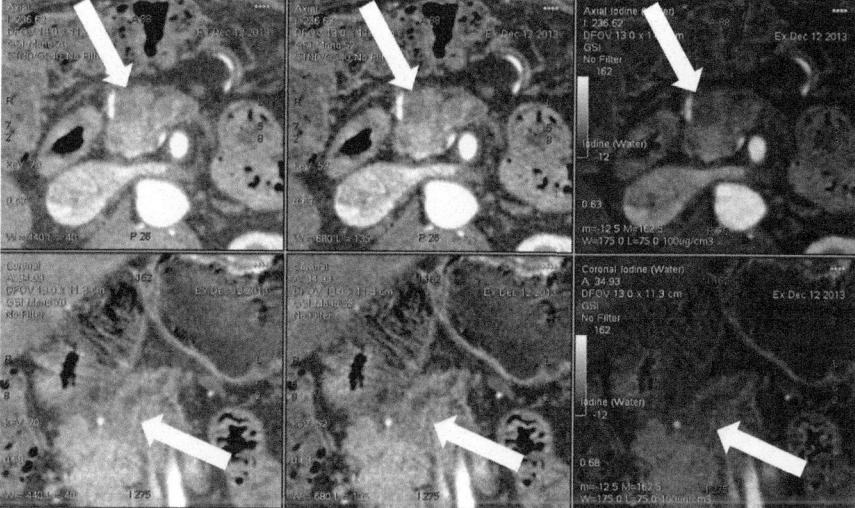

Fig. 6.2 A 61-year-old man with tiny pancreatic ductal adenocarcinoma. We have designed our DECT pancreatic parenchymal phase GSI server standard pancreatic carcinoma postprocessing "collage" to contain 70 keV (*left column*), 52 keV (*middle column*), iodine MD (*right column*), axial (*top*), and coronal (*bottom*) images. The 1.2 cm pancreatic adenocarcinoma in the anterior head region (*arrows*) is better visualized on the low energy 52 keV (*middle column*) images compared to the 70 keV (*left column*) images. The best definition of the margins is on the iodine image however. Our research has consistently shown the highest contrast to noise ratios on iodine MD images

6.2   Pancreas Adenocarcinoma

Pancreatic adenocarcinoma is a devastating disease and is projected by 2030 to be the second leading cause of cancer mortality [2–6]. Because survival can be improved with surgical intervention, particularly for small or lower stage tumors (Fig. 6.3), early detection and characterization is very important. Multiphasic multidetector CT (MDCT) plays a major role in this evaluation [4, 5], but there are still recognized shortcomings. Despite state of the art MDCT imaging, the sensitivity for detection of pancreatic ductal adenocarcinoma for lesions less than 2 cm is decreased [7].

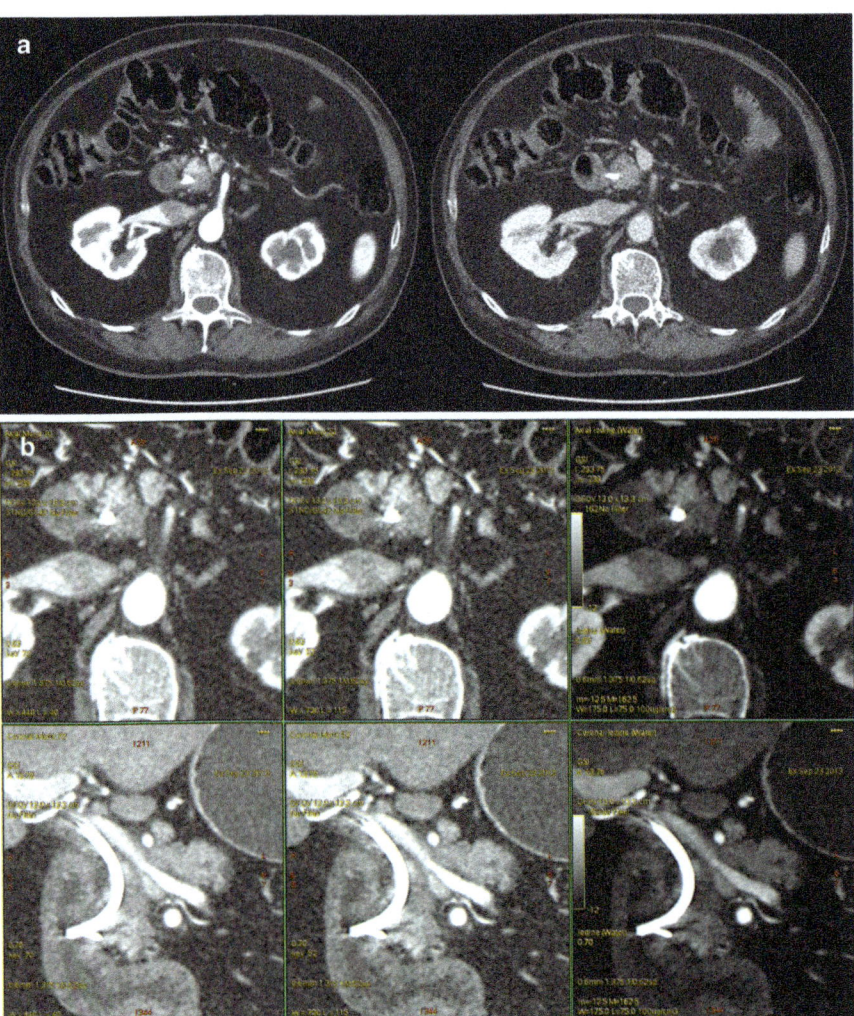

Fig. 6.3 A 60-year-old man with noncontour-altering isoattenuating pancreatic mass. (**a**) The lesion is not seen on single energy CT portal venous phase (*right*), but is visualized in the posterior pancreatic head region on dual energy pancreatic parenchymal phase (*left*). The lesion was also not well depicted on endoscopic ultrasound, and EUS FNA was negative for neoplasm on two occasions within 1 month after the DECT scan. (**b**) Pancreatic parenchymal phase GSI server "collage" with 70 keV (*left column*), 52 keV (*middle column*), iodine MD (*right column*), axial (*top*), and coronal (*bottom*) images reveal the tiny lesion in the mid aspect of the medial pancreatic head, adjacent to the stent. The margins are better depicted on the low energy and iodine images. This is borne out by the quantitative measurements on the 0.625 mm source images, which show higher absolute lesion contrast at low energies on (**c**). At resection, this lesion was a moderately differentiated pancreatic ductal adenocarcinoma, T3N0

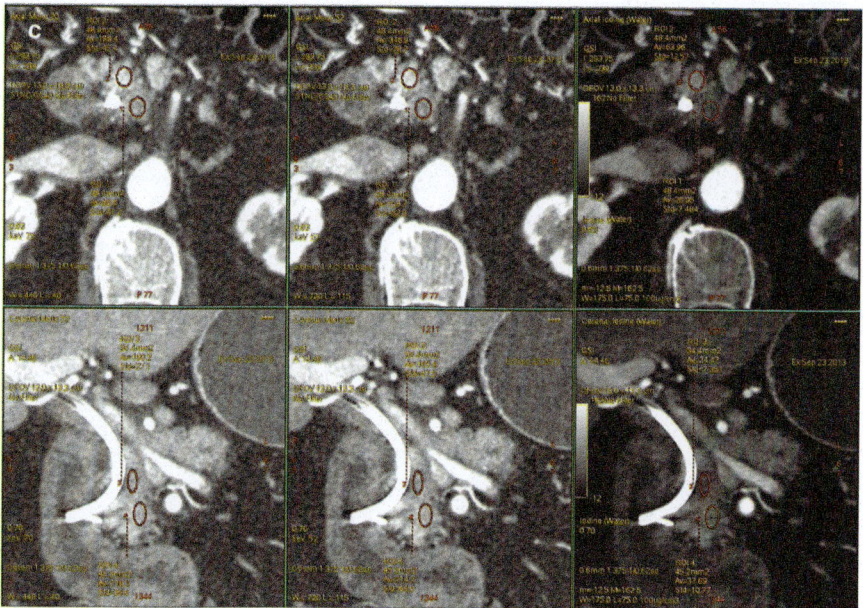

Fig. 6.3 (continued)

In addition, four to 27 % [8–10] of pancreatic cancers are isoattenuating (Fig. 6.4) to the adjacent pancreatic parenchyma, especially when small [9, 10]. These lesions may be discovered only by detection of secondary signs on imaging, such as segmental dilation of the pancreatic duct [10, 11].

Pancreatic adenocarcinoma is characteristically hypoattenuating relative to the adjacent parenchyma and is best depicted during the pancreatic parenchymal phase MDCT [12]. Complete assessment for vascular invasion and distant metastatic disease requires venous phase images [4, 13]; thus, state of the art single energy or standard pancreatic MDCT involves at least two acquisition image sets. Preliminary investigations utilizing dual energy CT [1, 14] and single energy low kVp imaging [15, 16] have demonstrated improved conspicuity of hypovascular pancreatic adenocarcinomas at lower viewing or acquisition energy levels. In our practice at present, DECT is acquired through the upper abdomen during the pancreatic parenchymal phase of a multiphasic exam, and single energy DECT is acquired through the abdomen and pelvis in portal venous phase. In efforts to reduce radiation exposure, Brook et al. [17] recently described a split bolus spectral DECT protocol that takes advantage of low (60 keV) energy DECT simulated monenergetic image viewing during hepatic venous phase while providing parenchymal attenuation values similar to a standard MDCT pancreatic parenchymal phase in patients with a variety of pancreatic lesions. Other investigators have reported improved detection and staging of focal pancreatic lesions using other types of images available only with DECT, such as iodine material density [18] images, or during novel modes of DECT

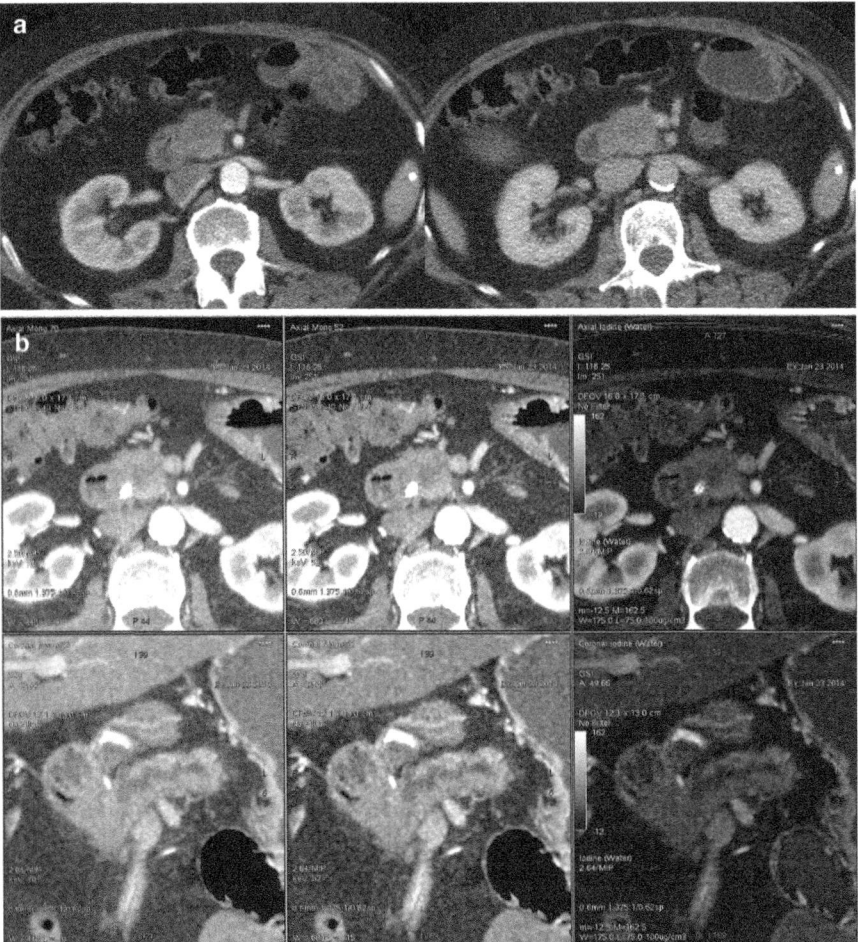

Fig. 6.4 A 64-year-old woman with isoattenuating pancreatic adenocarcinoma. (**a**) Multiphasic pancreatic single energy CT (pancreatic phase left, portal venous phase right) obtained at the referring hospital demonstrates a very poorly defined mass in the anterior pancreatic head. (**b**) Multiphasic pancreatic dual energy CT was performed. Pancreatic adenocarcinoma GSI server collage demonstrates the margin of the small mass in the anterior head region adjacent to the high density bile duct stent. Note the diminished artifact associated with the stent on the iodine MD images. The dilation of the main pancreatic duct to the level of the mass is best seen on the coronal images; this view is particularly helpful when the lesions are iso- or near-iosattenuating

image acquisition such as CT perfusion [19] and portal venography [20]. Although DECT acquisitions have been applied during a single venous phase [1], during the pancreatic parenchymal phase of a multiphasic abdominal protocol [14, 18], during a single split bolus single acquisition [17], and during alternative timing schemes, the principles resulting in production of advantageous image data apply no matter the timing. These will be described based on the category of dual energy image and the various types of pancreas neoplasms in more detail below.

6.3   Low Energy Applications

Macari et al. [1] first showed that conspicuity of pancreatic adenocarcinoma was greater using 80 kVp compared to blended 120 kVp images on dual source DECT obtained in portal venous phase. In this study, the weighting for the blended images was 0.3 for 80 kVp and 0.7 for 140 kVp. Chu et al. [21] identified that blended images with a weighting factor of 0.5 were preferred for evaluation of pancreatic diseases. Patel et al. [14] first showed the potential of rapid kV switching DECT acquired during pancreatic parenchymal phase to evaluate pancreatic adenocarcinoma lesion conspicuity in a cohort of 65 patients, and found a statistically significant increase of lesion contrast, a near doubling of the Hounsfield unit (HU) difference between tumoral and nontumoral tissue, on CNR-optimized keV images compared to the 70 keV image, the image energy typically used for routine PACS viewing (Fig. 6.5). The CNR-optimized keV calculation feature on the independent workstation and client server of the rapid kV switching DECT system workstation generates this value for each individual subject based on ROIs within tumoral and nontumoral tissue, and the mean optimized keV for the population in that early study was 52 keV. Note that with the rapid kV switching type of dual energy acquisition, there is no blended image and no generation of separate 80 and 140 kVp image sets for diagnosis. In a second study by the same group, a similar gain in conspicuity using low viewing energy was found for small pancreatic adenocarcinomas, an important and clinically relevant improvement, as smaller lesions might not alter the contour of the gland [18]. The use of lower simulated monoenergetic viewing energy (52 keV) in this study provided the best objective image quality measures (CNR, lesion contrast) for multiple readers. Also in that study, four of five lesions that were suspected clinically based on secondary findings of main pancreatic duct dilation were identified using low energy and iodine MD images combined with 70 keV [18] (Fig. 6.6). Others have also shown an improvement in pancreatic ductal adenocarcinoma detection by combining low keV imaging with a split bolus IV contrast administration technique [17] or by combining dsDECT 80 kVp images with a CT perfusion technique [19].

Improvement in lesion detectability was demonstrated by using monoenergetic 70 keV images compared to single energy images obtained at 120 kVp for a population of patients with small insulinomas (Fig. 6.7), where sensitivity for the preoperative diagnosis of insulinoma increased from 69 % with single energy CT to 87 % with DECT [22]. Not only important for evaluation of the primary pancreatic lesions, lower energy image viewing can enhance visualization of hypervascular liver lesions (Fig. 6.8). This has become important, because in clinical practice up to five metastases may be resected during initial debulking surgeries in patients with metastases from pancreatic neuroendocrine tumors. Other early experiences with low energy viewing of pancreatic endocrine neoplasms [23] and cystic pancreatic lesions [24] have been presented in abstracts. Visualization of nodules and

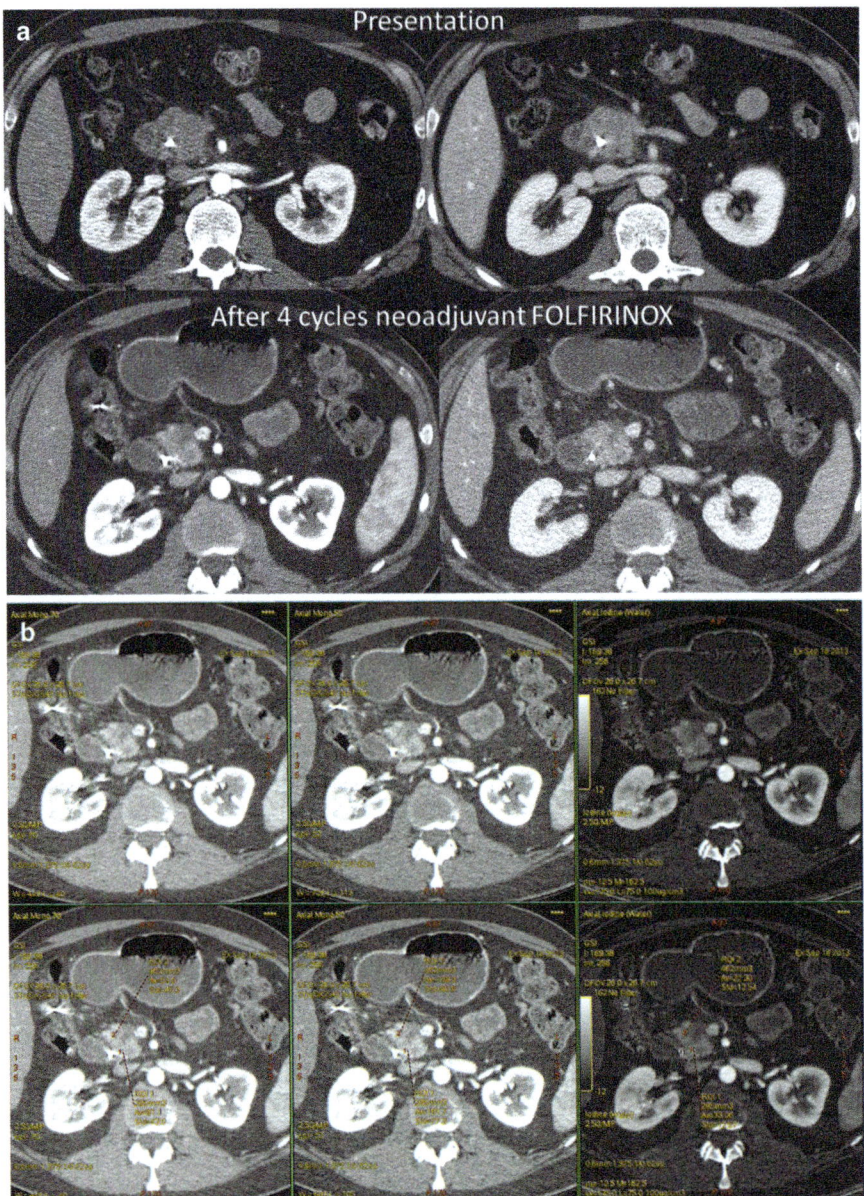

septations within cystic pancreas neoplasms (Fig. 6.9) was highest using CNR-optimized simulated monoenergetic keV (mean 51 keV for the population) and a gray-scale color filter compared to 70 keV without color filter, 70 keV with color filter, and CNR-optimized keV without filter [24]. Dual-energy technology appears promising for improved evaluation compared to single energy CT because of low viewing energy conspicuity gains for solid pancreatic lesions as well as improved visualization of complexity within cystic masses. Finally, creation of CT angiograms from the lower keV source images provides more robust surface rendered images for referring surgeons.

6.4   Material Specific Applications

Material specific images may enhance visualization for lesion detection or create opportunities to identify material contents of tumors (whether cystic or solid) or within complex pancreatic collections. Because iodine MD images typically have higher CNRs, small or isoattenuating pancreatic ductal adenocarcinomas and cystic pancreatic neoplasms may be best seen on these images. Review of iodine images yielded additional information in 50 % of cases in a population of 44 patients with focal pancreatic disease and proved useful for identifying the relationship of tumors to peripancreatic vessels [21]. In Lin's study of patients with small insulinomas the use of iodine MD images *together* with low energy images resulted in a further increase in detection from 87 % with DECT low energy image viewing alone and 87 % with iodine MD image viewing alone to 95.8 % [22] (see Fig. 6.7). In McNamara's study of patients with small pancreatic ductal adenocarcinomas, subjective lesion conspicuity and reader confidence were highest with iodine MD images [18]. The very low objectively measured image noise levels and statistically

---

Fig. 6.5 A 40-year-old man with small pancreatic ductal adenocarcinoma resected after four cycles of neoadjuvant therapy, portal vein graft required. (**a**) Pancreatic parenchymal phase (*left*) and portal venous phase (*right*) PACS images at presentation (*top*, single energy CT) and after neoadjuvant therapy with FOLFIRINOX (*bottom*, dual energy CT). A small heterogeneous hypovascular mass abuts the right margin of the superior mesenteric vein at the inferior pancreatic head level. Note that the lesion is not well distinguished on portal venous phase but is apparent on the pancreatic phase on the DECT. A biliary stent is in place. (**b**) Same patient DECT pancreatic parenchymal phase GSI server "collage" with 70 keV (*left column*), 52 keV (*middle column*) and iodine MD (*right column*) 2.5 mm images. The borders of the small mass are better seen on the 52 keV and iodine MD images, and the extent of involvement of the right lateral wall of the superior mesenteric vein (SMV) is more clearly seen. Volumetric regions of interest were drawn in the tumor and nontumoral tissue (*bottom row*) demonstrating the greater absolute lesion contrast on the 52 keV image compared to the 70 keV image. The 70 keV image is the simulated monoenergetic image energy that in our clinical practice most closely resembles images obtained at 120 kVp for single energy CT

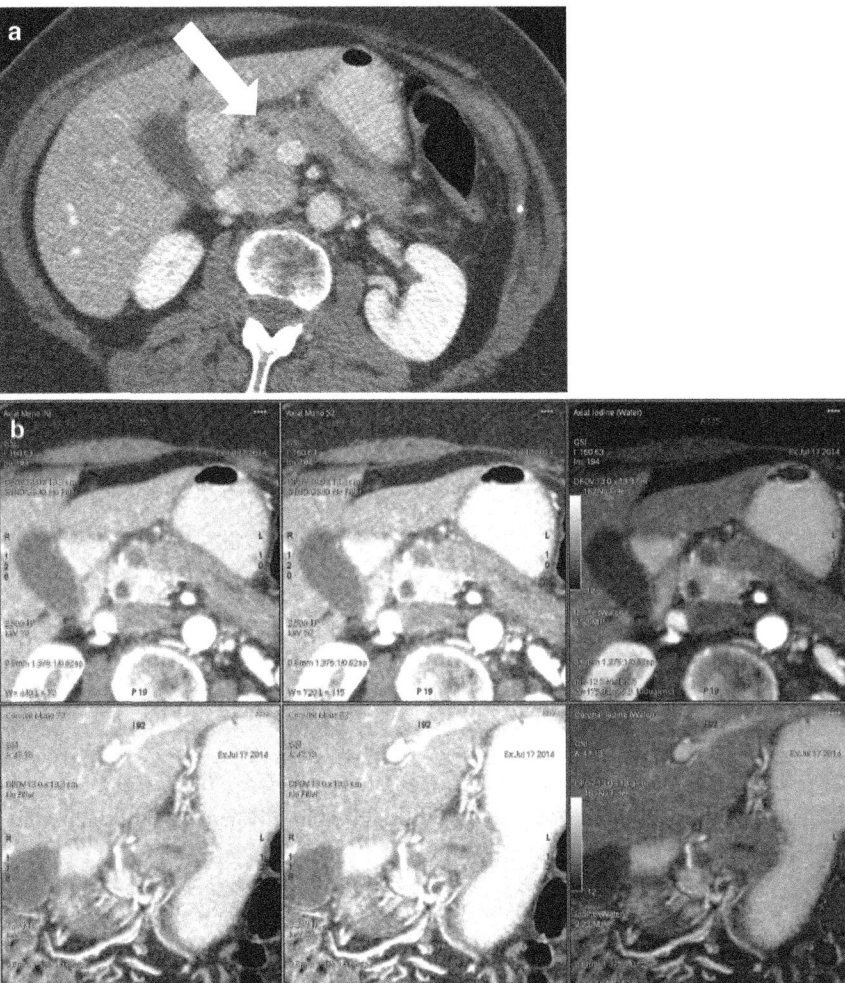

Fig. 6.6 A 72 year old woman with presenting with secondary signs of pancreatic cancer (**a**) Portal venous phase single energy CT image obtained at the referring hospital demonstrates dilation of the pancreatic duct in the tail/body region. There is slight heterogeneity in the anterior neck (*arrow*). The duct was not dilated downstream (towards the papilla) from this point. (**b**) Multiphasic pancreatic DECT was obtained for further evaluation. GSI server standard pancreatic carcinoma postprocessing "collage" with 70 keV (*left column*), 52 keV (*middle column*), and iodine MD (*right column*) 2.5 mm reformatted images demonstrate the tiny round subcentimeter pancreatic adenocarcinoma at the site of duct cut off, better seen on the coronal image (*bottom row*). There is marked differential enhancement of the gland upstream in the body and tail region from downstream in the head region. The patient underwent EUS fine needle aspiration biopsies which were negative, demonstrating only chronic inflammation. (**c**) Same patient 12 weeks later. GSI server collage demonstrates that the hypovascular mass in the pancreatic neck has now grown to greater than 2 cm. The relationship of the mass to the main pancreatic duct is better seen on the coronal images. (**d**) On the same multiphasic CT exam, the single energy CT portal venous phase images revealed a well-circumscribed hypodensity in the interlobar region of the liver (*arrow*) that was new and therefore highly suspicious for distant metastatic disease. (**e**) GSI server collage through the level of the suspicious liver lesion reveals rim-like enhancement, indicating metastatic disease. This image presentation uses a gray scale color "perfusion" filter to enhance visualization of hyperenhancing lesions such as hepatocellular carcinomas or metastatic gastrointestinal stromal tumors

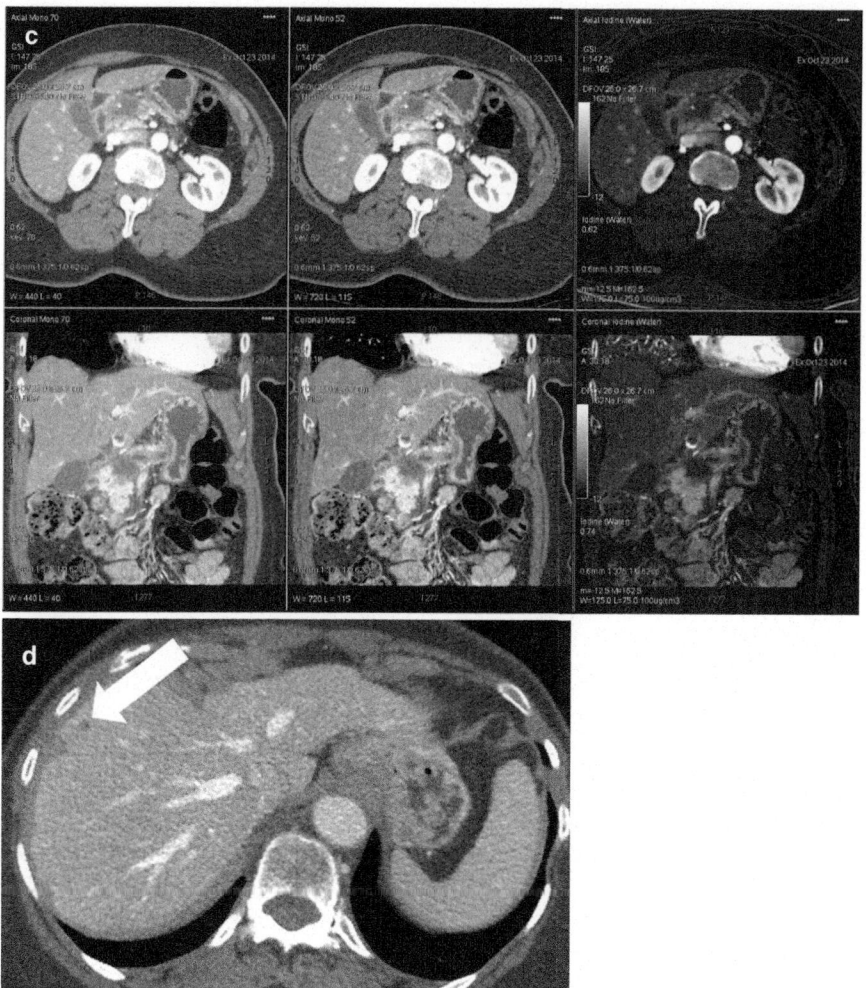

Fig. 6.6   (continued)

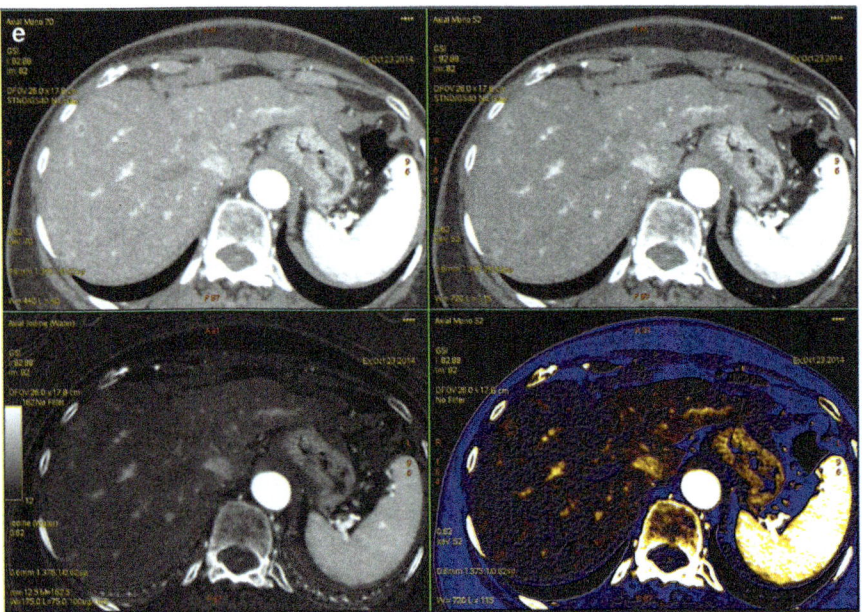

Fig. 6.6 (continued)

greater CNR likely contributed to the favorable rating of these images (see Fig. 6.2). It is important to point out that the ability to create complimentary iodine MD and lower viewing energy images with the same DECT acquisition distinguishes this method from simple image acquisition utilizing a lower tube voltage single energy CT, which has been previously shown to enhance visualization of focal pancreatic lesions in phantom [16] and patient [15, 25] studies.

Iodine MD images represent only one type of material density image available using DECT. Virtual unenhanced images (discussed in greater detail elsewhere in other chapters) typically refer to water MD images that are created through three-material decomposition using dual source dual energy scanners or through material basis pair decomposition using rapid kV switching scanners. National Institute of Standards and Technology (NIST) x-ray attenuation curves are available for other human tissue materials such as blood and mucin, therefore, with dual-energy CT a potential exists to evaluate the contents of focal pancreatic lesions to differentiate mucin-containing cystic pancreatic neoplasms from other pancreatic cystic lesions (Fig. 6.10), or to identify blood versus residual enhancing pancreas in necrotic pancreatic collections. The use of dedicated metal artifact reduction algorithms, or simply viewing iodine MD or 140 keV images provides more optimal viewing of the pancreas around metallic bile duct stents or surgical clips that may be present from prior hepatic or pancreatic resections, similar to reduction of metal artifacts around joint prostheses [26].

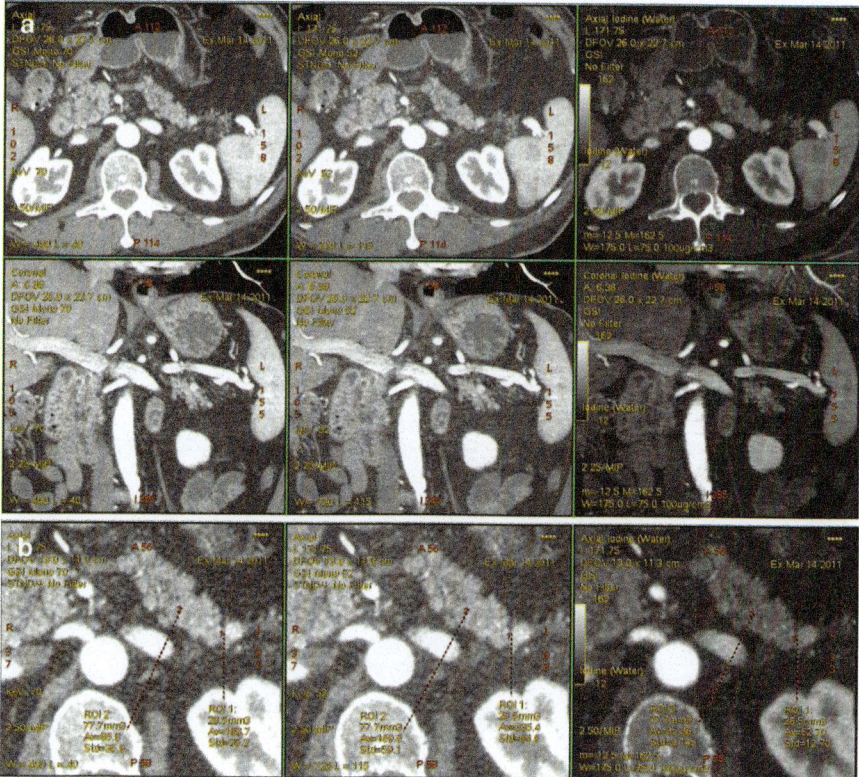

Fig. 6.7 A 66-year-old man with tiny pancreatic endocrine neoplasm. (**a**) DECT pancreatic parenchymal phase GSI server standard pancreatic carcinoma postprocessing "collage" with 70 keV (*left column*), 52 keV (*middle column*), iodine MD (*right column*), axial (*top*), and coronal (*bottom*) images work well for evaluation of hyperenhancing solid lesions as well. The subcentimeter hypervascular mass in the pancreatic tail region is well seen on both axial 2.5 mm (*top*) and coronal 2.25 mm (*bottom*) reformatted images. (**b**) Same level axial images with smaller field-of-view. ROI analysis again shows that there is greater tumor to nontumoral tissue difference at low energy (*middle*) compared to the 70 keV image (*left*)

6.5 Isoattenuating Focal Pancreatic Masses

Because small, noncontour-altering isoattenuating lesions remain a challenge for state of the art single energy MDCT, one real opportunity for DECT is to identify these types of lesions (see Figs. 6.3 and 6.4). This increased detectability provided by DECT was shown in the multireader study by McNamara et al. [18], where four of five subjects who did not have an identifiable or measurable mass on prospective clinical interpretations using only the 70 keV images had tumors identified on lower (52 keV) energy and iodine MD images combined with the 70 keV images. A similar phenomenon was described by Lin et al. [22], where nontypical (iso- or

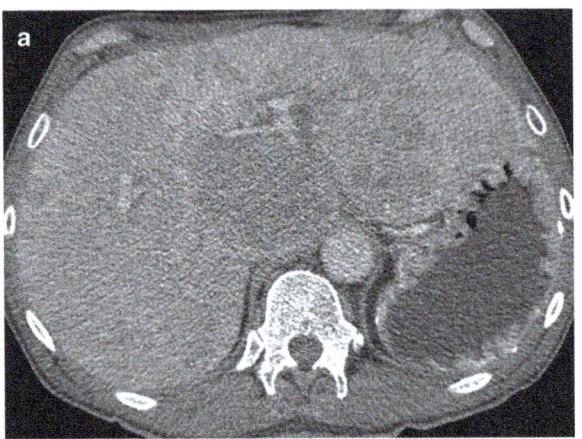

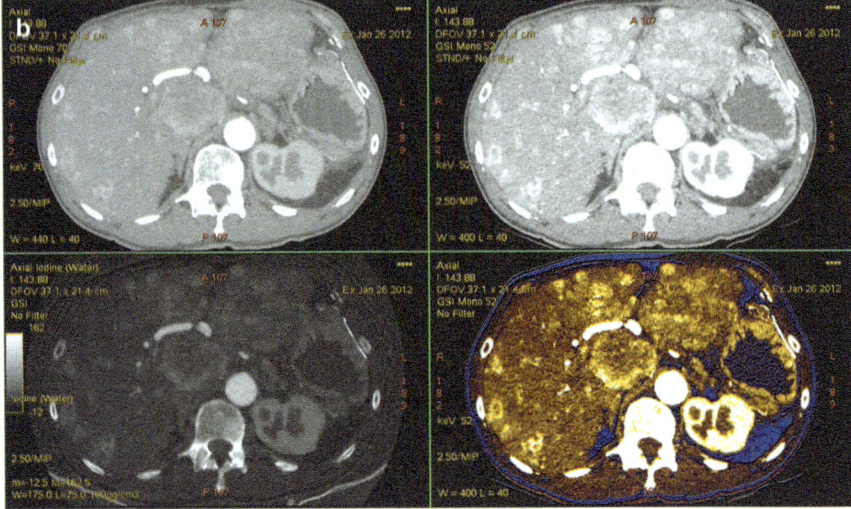

Fig. 6.8 A 61-year-old man with advanced pancreatic endocrine neoplasm. (**a**) Portal venous phase single energy axial CT image demonstrates large caudate hypovascular mass, with additional disease seen in the lateral and anterior segments. With pancreatic endocrine neoplasms, liver metastases are better depicted on either pancreatic parenchymal or in this case late hepatic arterial phase since the patient had undergone distal pancreatectomy. (**b**) Same patient DECT acquisition in late hepatic arterial phase. We designed the GSI server collage highlighting hyperenhancing lesions to contain 70 keV (*upper left*), 52 keV (*upper right*), iodine (-H$_2$O) material density (*lower left*), and 52 keV with gray scale color "perfusion" images. The latter readily depicts the metastatic tumor burden in the liver, much greater than that seen on portal venous phase. Although not necessary for this patient with extensive metastatic disease, this visualization technique can be very helpful for rapid assessment of smaller lesions

hypoattenuating) small pancreatic endocrine neoplasms not detected with 70 keV were seen with combined low energy and iodine MD images. Additionally, the difficulty in detection of isoattenuating tumors may be addressed with DECT perfusion pancreas imaging as described by Klauss et al. [19]. In their study, all 24

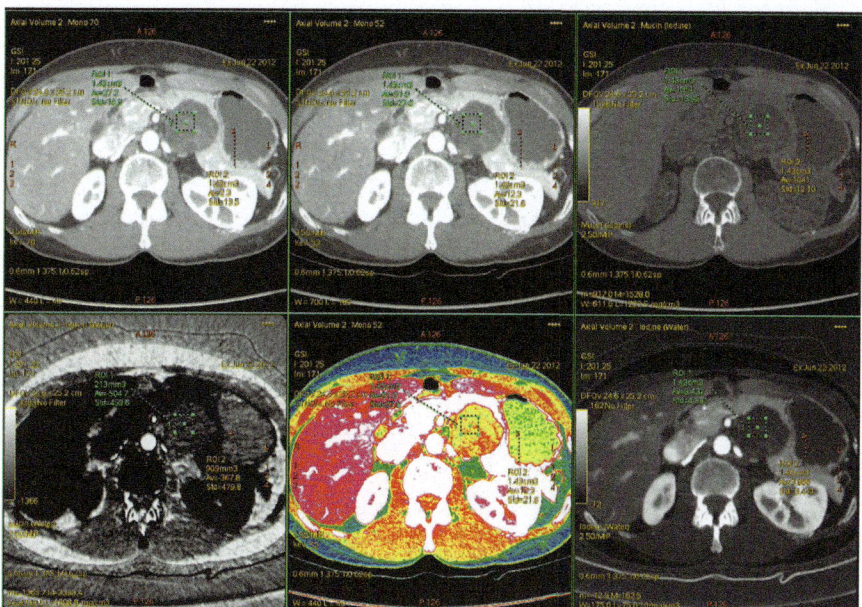

Fig. 6.9 A 40-year-old woman with incidental discovery of a cystic pancreatic lesion discovered during renal stone evaluation. Multiphasic dual energy pancreatic CT was performed. GSI server collage optimized to evaluate pancreatic cystic lesions contains 70 keV (*upper left*), 52 keV (*upper middle*), mucin (-iodine) material density (*upper right*), material density (*lower left*), 52 keV with gray scale color "French" filter (*middle bottom*), and iodine (-H_2O) (*right bottom*) images. Note that in this mucinous cystic neoplasm which contained dysplastic cells on pathologic evaluation after resection, there are multiple septations and nodules better visualized by the red coloration compared to the yellow mucin background on the "French" filter low energy image. The mucin in the cyst has a slightly higher quantitative value than the water in the stomach on the mucin (-iodine) MD image; on the mucin (-H_2O) image the value in the lesion is more negative than the water in the stomach

pancreatic ductal adenocarcinomas were detected using perfusion maps, whereas four (20 %) had no mass visible on either pancreatic parenchymal or portal venous phase conventional single energy MDCT.

6.6   Post Processing and Image Visualization

Using DECT software, it is possible to view the lower keV images and 70 keV images side by side with iodine material density (MD) images, a practice which also enhances lesion detection due to the lower contrast to noise ratios (CNR) of iodine MD images [27]. Color coding or iodine threshold imaging techniques can potentially help radiologists rapidly assess images, particularly for oncology patients. While these techniques have been described largely for other abdominal organs and disease processes, applications in the pancreas, such as for depiction of cystic pancreatic masses are usable today. The ability to create, view, and quantify lower

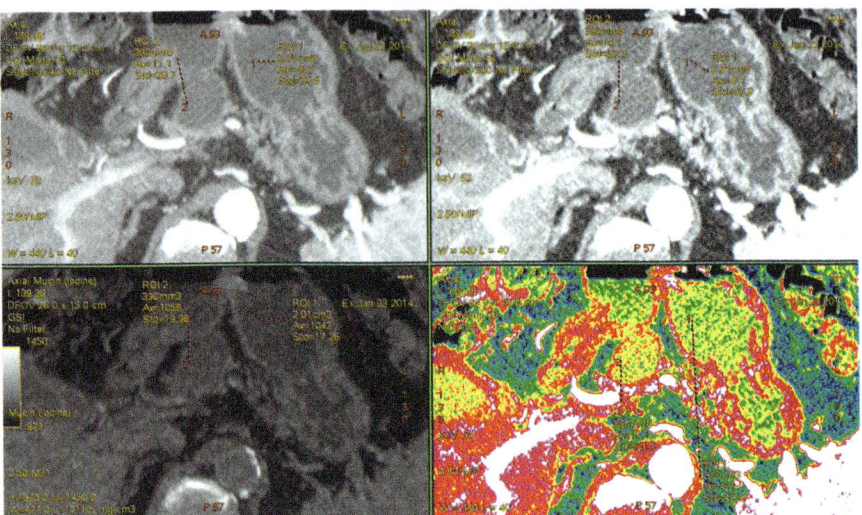

Fig. 6.10 A 77-year-old man with side branch IP MN. Pancreatic parenchymal phase DECT GSI server collage with 70 keV (*upper left*), 52 keV (*upper right*), mucin (-iodine) material density (*lower left*), and 52 keV with gray scale color "French" filter (*lower right*) images. There is a similar appearance of cyst contents and water in the stomach on the simulated monoenergetic images. However, the quantification is slightly different on the mucin (-iodine) material density image, and the colorization shows that the contents of the cyst are clearly different than that of the gastric water. Although the EUSFNA aspirate revealed a CEA of 241,000, this lesion was a benign side branch type IPMN upon pathologic inspection following central pancreatectomy

energy images, iodine and other material density images, and multimaterial decomposition images using dual energy CT provides advantages in clinical practice compared to low kVp single energy CT abdominal imaging techniques alone. In several studies radiologists have demonstrated subjective preference for blended images or simulated monoenergetic images at 70 or 77 keV [17, 18] which appear similar to 120 kVp single energy CT images, but the highest objective image quality measures (such as tumoral to nontumoral contrast difference, and contrast to noise ratios) as well as subjective lesion conspicuity and reader confidence are found for the low energy and iodine DECT image sets. Furthermore, near perfect to very high multi-reader kappa statistic values for DECT image analysis by practitioners with variable levels of experience [18] indicate that these types or images are ready to be utilized in daily clinical practice. The use of postprocessing to enhance daily workflow is important to continue to investigate, however, seamless incorporation into existing PACS and rapid selection of optimum postprocessing protocols (Fig. 6.11) for individual patient requirements is absolutely mandatory.

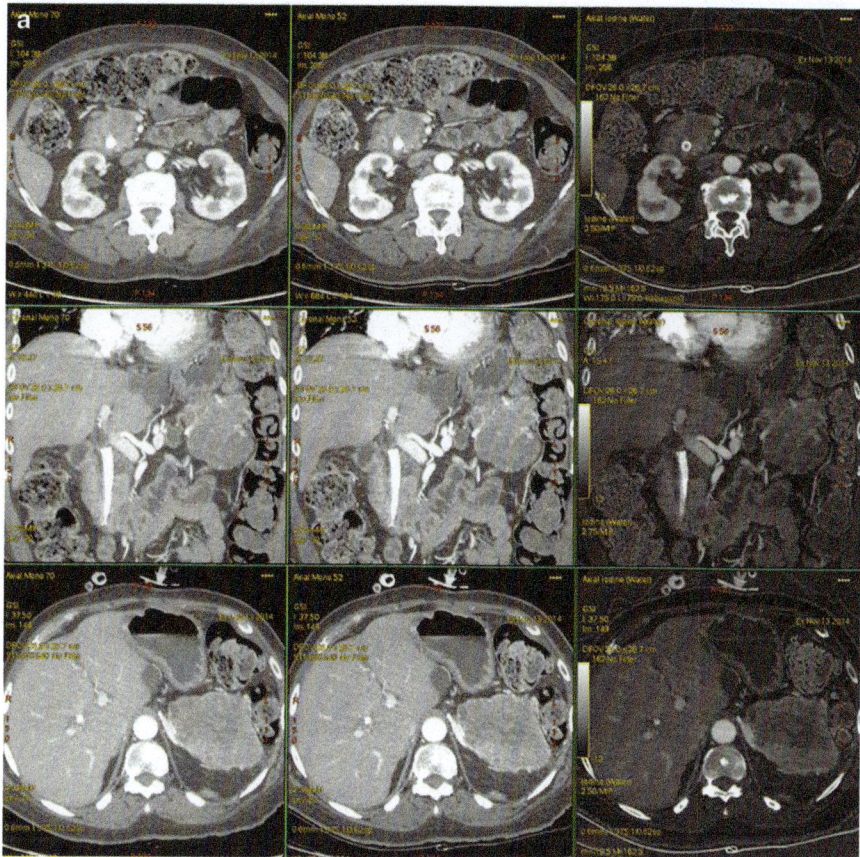

Fig. 6.11 A 73-year-old woman with pancreatic head adenocarcinoma and pancreatic tail serous cystadenoma. (**a**) Pancreatic parenchymal phase GSI server pancreatic adenocarcinoma "collage" with 70 keV (*left column*), 52 keV (*middle column*), iodine MD (*right column*), axial (*top*), and coronal (*bottom*) images at the level of the pancreatic head adenocarcinoma (*top* and *middle row*) and pancreatic tail serous cystadenoma (axial images *bottom row*) demonstrate the better depiction of the hypovascular adenocarcinoma at low energy and on iodine MD images. The internal architecture of the microcystic lesion is best seen on the iodine images as well. (**b**) Applying the "pancreatic cyst" GSI server "collage" to the serous cystadenoma, the complexity of the tiny cysts renders the lesion more solid appearing, similar to the liver parenchyma on the 52 keV images with gray scale color "French" filter (*bottom right*)

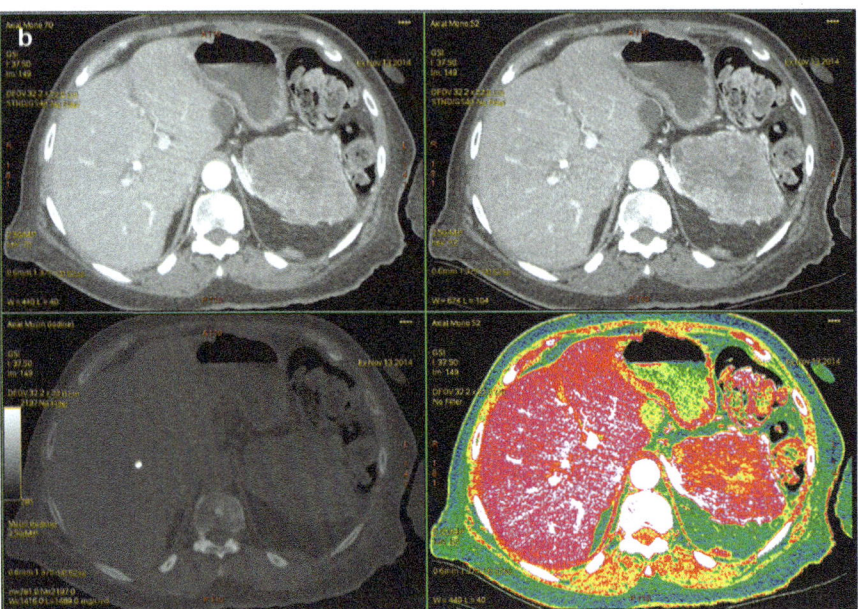

Fig. 6.11 (continued)

References

1. Macari M, Spieler B, Kim D et al (2010) Dual-source dual-energy MDCT of pancreatic adeno-carcinoma: initial observations with data generated at 80 kVp and simulated weighted-average 120 kVp. AJR Am J Roentgenol 194:W27–W32
2. American Cancer Society (2013) Cancer facts and figures 2013. American Cancer Society, Atlanta
3. Howlader N, Noone AM, Krapcho M et al SEER cancer statistics review, 1975–2010. National Cancer Institute, Bethesda. http://seer.cancer.gov/csr/1975_2010/, Based on November 2012 SEER data submission, posted to the SEER web site, April 2013. Surveillance, Epidemiology, and End Results Program
4. Callery MP, Chang KJ, Fishman EK et al (2009) Pretreatment assessment of resectable and borderline resectable pancreatic cancer: expert consensus statement. Ann Surg Oncol 16: 1727–1733
5. Tamm EP, Silverman PM, Charnsangavej C et al (2003) Diagnosis, staging, and surveillance of pancreatic cancer. AJR Am J Roentgenol 180(5):1311–1323
6. Rahib L, Smith BD, Aizenberg R et al (2014) Projecting cancer incidence and deaths to 2030: the unexpected burden of thyroid, liver, and pancreas cancers in the United States. Cancer Res 74(11):2913–2921
7. Bronstein YL, Loyer EM, Kaur H et al (2004) Detection of small pancreatic tumors with mul-tiphasic helical CT. AJR Am J Roentgenol 182(3):619–623
8. Prokesch RW, Chow LC, Beaulieu CF et al (2002) Isoattenuating pancreatic adenocarcinoma at multi-detector row CT: secondary signs. Radiology 224:764–768
9. Kim JH, Park SH, Yu ES et al (2010) Visually isoattenutating pancreatic adenocarcinoma at dynamic-enhanced CT: frequency, clinical and pathologic characteristics, and diagnosis at imaging examinations. Radiology 257(1):87–96

10. Yoon SH, Lee JM, Cho JY et al (2011) Small (≤20 mm) pancreatic adenocarcinomas: analysis of enhancement patterns and secondary signs with multiphasic multidetector CT. Radiology 259:442–452

11. Gangi S, Fletcher JG, Nathan MA et al (2004) Time interval between abnormalities seen on CT and the clinical diagnosis of pancreatic cancer: retrospective review of CT scans obtained before diagnosis. AJR Am J Roentgenol 182:897–903

12. Lu DS, Vedantham S, Krasny RM et al (1996) Two-phase helical CT for pancreatic tumors: pancreatic versus hepatic phase enhancement of tumor, pancreas, and vascular structures. Radiology 199:697–701

13. Fletcher JG, Wiersema MJ, Farrell MA et al (2003) Pancreatic malignancy: value of arterial, pancreatic, and hepatic phase imaging with multi-detector row CT. Radiology 229(1):81–90

14. Patel BN, Thomas JV, Lockhart ME et al (2013) Single–source dual–energy spectral multidetector CT of pancreatic adenocarcinoma: optimization of energy level viewing significantly increases lesion contrast. Clin Radiol 68(2):148–154

15. Marin D, Nelson RC, Barnhart H et al (2010) Detection of pancreatic tumors, image quality, and radiation dose during the pancreatic parenchymal phase: effect of low-tube-voltage, high-tube-current CT technique-preliminary results. Radiology 256:450–459

16. Holm J, Louizou L, Albiin N et al (2012) Low tube voltage CT for improved detection of pancreatic cancer: detection threshold for small, simulated lesions. BMC Med Imaging 12:20

17. Brook OR, Gourtsoyianni S, Brook A et al (2013) Split-bolus spectral multidetector CT of the pancreas: assessment of radiation dose and tumor conspicuity. Radiology 269:139–148

18. McNamara MM, Little MD, Alexander LF et al (2015) Abdom Imaging 40(5):1230–1240. doi: 10.1007/s00261-014-0274-y. PMID: 25331567

19. Klauss M, Stiller W, Pahn G et al (2013) Dual-energy perfusion-CT of pancreatic adenocarcinoma. Eur J Radiol 82:208–214

20. Zhao L, He W, Li J et al (2012) Improving image quality in portal venography with spectral CT imaging. Eur J Radiol 81:1677–1681

21. Chu AJ, Lee JM, Lee YJ et al (2012) Dual-source, dual-energy multidetector CT for the evaluation of pancreatic tumours. Br J Radiol 85:e891–e898

22. Lin XZ, Wu ZY, Tao R (2012) Dual energy spectral CT imaging of insulinoma-value in preoperative diagnosis compared with conventional multi-detector CT. Eur J Radiol 81:2487–2494

23. Balachandran A, Bhosale P, Fox P et al (2013) Primary comparison of contrast to noise ratios for pancreatic neuroendocrine neoplasms for dual-energy CT versus 120 kVp single-energy CT. ARRS Annual Meeting, Washington, DC

24. Cunningham J, Patel B, Thomas JV et al (2011) Spectral MDCT analysis of cystic pancreatic lesions: can dual energy acquisition and spectral viewing aid in detection of septations and nodules? Scientific paper presented at the ARRS Annual Meeting, Chicago

25. Marin D, Boll DT, Mileto A et al (2014) State of the art: dual-energy CT of the abdomen. Radiology 271(2):327–342

26. Pessis E, Campagna R, Sverzut JM et al (2013) Metal artifacts reduction using monochromatic images from spectral CT: evaluation of pedicle screws in patients with scoliosis. Eur J Radiol pii: S0720-048X(13)00110-1. doi:10.1016/j.ejrad.2013.02.024

27. Morgan DE (2014) Dual energy CT of the abdomen. Abdom Imaging 39:108–134

Dual Energy CT in Gastrointestinal Tumors

7

Paul Apfaltrer

7.1 Introduction

Radiological imaging of the gastrointestinal tract provides useful diagnostic information regarding a wide variety of benign and malignant tumors. Although MRI, due to its superior soft tissue contrast options, is considered superior for characterization of various soft tissue lesions, in clinical practice computed tomography (CT) often will be the first and only imaging technique. CT has still an important role in the detection and diagnosis of gastrointestinal tumors and represents clinical practice for evaluating adjacent organ invasion, distant metastasis, and peritoneal seeding. A recent development in CT has been the introduction of dual-source technology. On such CT systems, two X-ray tubes can be operated at different tube potentials, making "dual-energy scanning" possible [1]. Dual-energy CT (DECT) imaging implies the acquisition of CT data with two different X-ray spectra, and it can be obtained through several commercially available hardware platforms [2]. DECT applications are based on two distinct capabilities: material differentiation and material identification and quantification. Material differentiation means obtaining material-specific images with separation, and material identification and quantification mean accurate assessment of the presence and amount of, for example, iodine in a target lesion [3].

These foregoing technical advances in CT imaging, in particular, the possibility of DECT imaging, yielded to clear advantages in tumor detection, lesion characterization, and evaluation of response to therapy in oncological imaging. The technology opens up the possibility of advanced assessment and documentation of therapy response by concurrent quantification of tumor size and iodine uptake and proposes a unifying solution to the issues related to multiphase scanning, contrast medium

P. Apfaltrer, MD
Department of Biomedical Imaging and Image-Guided Therapy,
Medical University of Vienna, Vienna, Austria
e-mail: paul.apfaltrer@meduniwien.ac.at

© Springer International Publishing Switzerland 2015
C.N. De Cecco et al. (eds.), *Dual Energy CT in Oncology*,
DOI 10.1007/978-3-319-19563-6_7

95

volume, and radiation dose [3, 4]. The combination of low-energy images and iodine as well as the different applications of postprocessed DECT images has the potential to change the way oncologic patients are assessed and monitored. The raw data derived from DECT may be mathematically manipulated to generate postprocessed datasets, including material-specific iodine, virtual monochromatic (VMC), and virtual nonenhanced (VNE) images [5]. Because the behavior of iodine at different energies is known, iodine may be extracted from an image to generate a set of simulated unenhanced images, thus eliminate the need for separate unenhanced datasets with consequently reduced radiation dose and examination time for the patients [5].

The potential applications of DECT when evaluating the abdomen are numerous. Clinical applications seek to use the technical characteristics of DECT and recent developments toward quantitative and functional imaging, particularly in the context of material-specific imaging, underline the increasing importance of DECT in oncology [2]. However, studies using DECT in radiological imaging of the gastrointestinal tract are rare, as until recently, the main two focuses for abdominal oncological imaging using DECT were the detection and characterization of focal liver lesions and second oncological imaging of pancreatic cancer. Recent studies suggest that DECT has the potential to improve the differentiation between benign and malignant tissue in gastrointestinal cancers, but more prospective clinical evidence will be needed in this context.

7.2   Esophageal and Gastric Malignancy

Esophageal carcinomas are mostly asymptomatic in early stages and most patients are referred to diagnostic procedures at an advanced stage [6]. However, some patients may exhibit dysphagia, bleeding, or other symptoms. Occasionally, early esophageal cancers can be detected by serendipity or by screening of asymptomatic patients in high-risk groups. Accurate staging is crucial to assess the therapeutic regimen and the possibility for cure by operative tumor removal [6]. It is of importance to exclude distant metastases and to ensure a response to radiation therapy and chemotherapy if these are used in a curative approach before surgery. Regardless of the morphology of the tumor, CT typically reveals marked circumferential thickening of the esophageal wall. Infiltrating carcinomas are usually manifested on barium studies by irregular luminal narrowing with mucosal nodularity, ulceration, and abrupt, shelf-like proximal and distal borders [7]. The standard diagnostic tools in this tumor entity are endoscopic ultrasonography (EUS) for local assessment of the T and N statuses and CT for additional searching for distant metastases. Biopsy remains the gold standard for identifying malignant disease and T staging relies on the histopathologic examination of resected tissue [6]. Squamous cell carcinomas tend to be located in the upper or mid-esophagus, whereas adenocarcinomas predominantly are located in the distal esophagus and have a marked tendency to invade the gastric cardia and fundus. EUS as well as integrated PET/CT with 2-[18F]-fluoro-2-deoxy-D-glucose (FDG) has emerged as an important and recommended part of routine staging of patients with esophageal cancer in international guidelines [8–10]. Knowledge of tumor extent and its relationship with vascular structures is important for treatment planning. Ongoing research is performed if

DECT may also help confirm the morphologic and enhancement characteristics of esophageal cancer. In particular, DECT may be used for direct visualization of iodine uptake within tumor in color-coded fashion, which may allow a reliable quantification of tumor enhancement.

Gastric carcinoma is one of the most common tumors and generally has a poor prognosis. It is classified according to histologic characteristics [6] with two major subgroups of microscopic growth pattern, the so-called intestinal type and the nonintestinal or diffuse type [6, 11]. The extent of stomach wall invasion by the tumor spread to the lymph nodes and the presence of distal organ metastases determine the stage of the tumor [12]. Gastric adenocarcinoma usually arises from the distal esophagus or the esophagogastric junction and first spreads locally, mostly through the gastric wall. Standard diagnostic tools in the assessment of gastric carcinomas are EUS and CT or staging laparoscopy [6]. Both CT and PET are useful for assessment of treatment response following preoperative chemotherapy and for detection of recurrence after surgical resection [12]. MRI, despite its better soft tissue contrast and direct multiplanar imaging capability, is less preferred than CT due to prolonged scanning time and higher cost [12]. Perfusion CT has been proposed for measurement of angiogenesis and tumor perfusion [13, 14] Preliminary studies with perfusion CT of gastric cancer have shown that the blood volume is significantly increased in gastric cancer compared to that of normal stomach mucosa [12, 15]. As DECT allows quantification of intravenously injected iodinated contrast media in tumors, and therefore may be considered as a surrogate marker for perfusion and tumor vascularity, DECT may also provide additional information for preoperative staging and assessment of treatment response, respectively (Fig. 7.1). However, studies validating the usefulness of DECT in for individualized treatment of gastric cancer are eagerly awaited.

Gastrointestinal stromal tumors (GIST) represent an extremely rare neoplasm which is increasingly recognized as a distinct tumor entity of soft tissue tumors. The majority of these gastrointestinal tumors are located in the stomach and small intestine and compose 1–3 % of malignant gastrointestinal tumors [16, 17]. Metastases are most common in the liver, mesentery, and peritoneum. On imaging, small GISTs are mostly well-defined solid mass with homogenous enhancement; larger tumors may show areas of hemorrhage, cystic/necrotic areas, and heterogeneous enhancement (Fig. 7.2). After contrast administration neovascularity may be seen within the tumor [18]. Therapeutic options for GIST include radical surgery for primary tumors and targeted therapy with tyrosine kinase inhibitors imatinib or sunitinib for metastatic disease [19–21]. Radiologic appearances can change drastically after therapy and knowledge of such imaging features is beneficial in managing these patients. With the recent introduction of targeted therapy for imatinib, clinical management and prognosis of GIST patients have improved significantly. Response to imatinib is characterized by decreased enhancement, resolution of the enhancing tumor nodules, and a decrease in tumor neovascularity, and these changes are usually seen within 1 month of initiation of chemotherapy [18]. Since the introduction of these molecularly targeted drugs, there has been increasing concern about the use of traditional tumor response criteria (e.g., WHO or RECIST), as several studies have indicated that response to treatment is not equivalent to a change in tumor size [22, 23]. Choi et al. have proposed the measurement of CT attenuation values as a potential indicator of GIST response in patients undergoing targeted therapy.

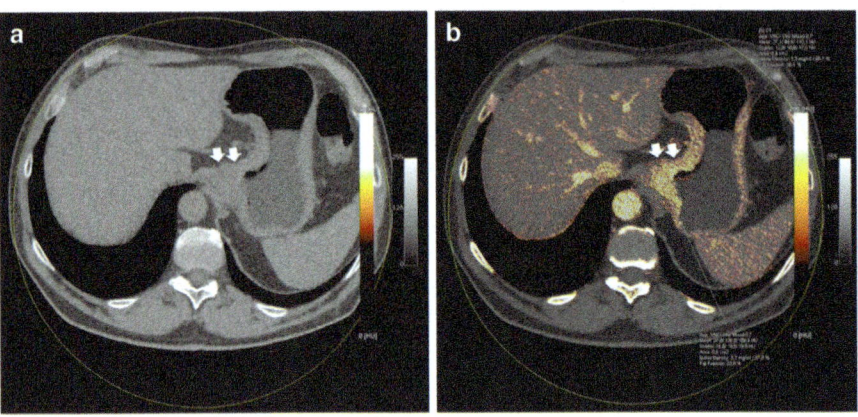

Fig. 7.1 A 69-year-old male with biopsy-proven adenocarcinoma of the stomach shown on axial non-contrast-enhanced CT images (**a**) and fused color-coded iodine maps (**b**) (*arrows*). The DECT shows excellent intralesional iodine uptake within tumor in color-coded fashion, which makes a reliable quantification of enhancement. The region of interest displays higher contrast enhancement and iodine density within the tumor (126.9 HU; 5.7 mg/ml) compared to normal gastric wall (84.5 HU; 3.3 mg/ml), respectively (**b**)

According to the Choi criteria, tumor density is determined by drawing regions of interest (ROI) circumscribing the margin of the tumor on portal venous-phase CT images [19, 24, 25]. Choi et al. have demonstrated that a decrease in tumor size of >10 % or a decrease in tumor density of >15 % had a sensitivity of 97 % and a specificity of 100 % in detecting patients with good response to treatment with imatinib evaluated by PET-CT in metastatic GIST [18, 26]. Decreased density of responding GIST on CT pathologically correlates with the development of tumor necrosis on histopathology and cystic or myxoid degeneration; however, GIST response may result in increased density because of intratumoral hemorrhage, which is a rare but well-known effect observed during imatinib therapy [19, 27, 28] (Fig. 7.2).

DECT allows selective quantification and visualization of iodine-related attenuation (IRA) differences [19] which facilitates the generation of VNE CT images and can be used to improve the lesion conspicuity [29]. As previously described, VNE CT data calculated from DECT might potentially eliminate the need for acquisition of a separate unenhanced dataset, which could result in a considerable decrease in radiation exposure to patients [19] (Fig. 7.2). Several studies on abdominal (renal and liver) DECT have shown good correlation between VNE and TNE CT Series [30–32].

Fig. 7.2 True nonenhanced images (TNE) single-energy CT (**a**) and DECT (**b–e**) of a patient with metastatic GIST. TNE (**a**) and virtual nonenhanced images (**b**) similarly demonstrate intrametastatic hemorrhage of the liver metastasis in the left liver lobe (*arrowheads*). Virtual 120 kV image (**c**) is unable to differentiate between the intrametastatic hemorrhage and enhancing parts of the metastasis. Iodine map (**e**) as well as the fused iodine map (**d**) demonstrates the enhancing and well-perfused parts of the metastasis

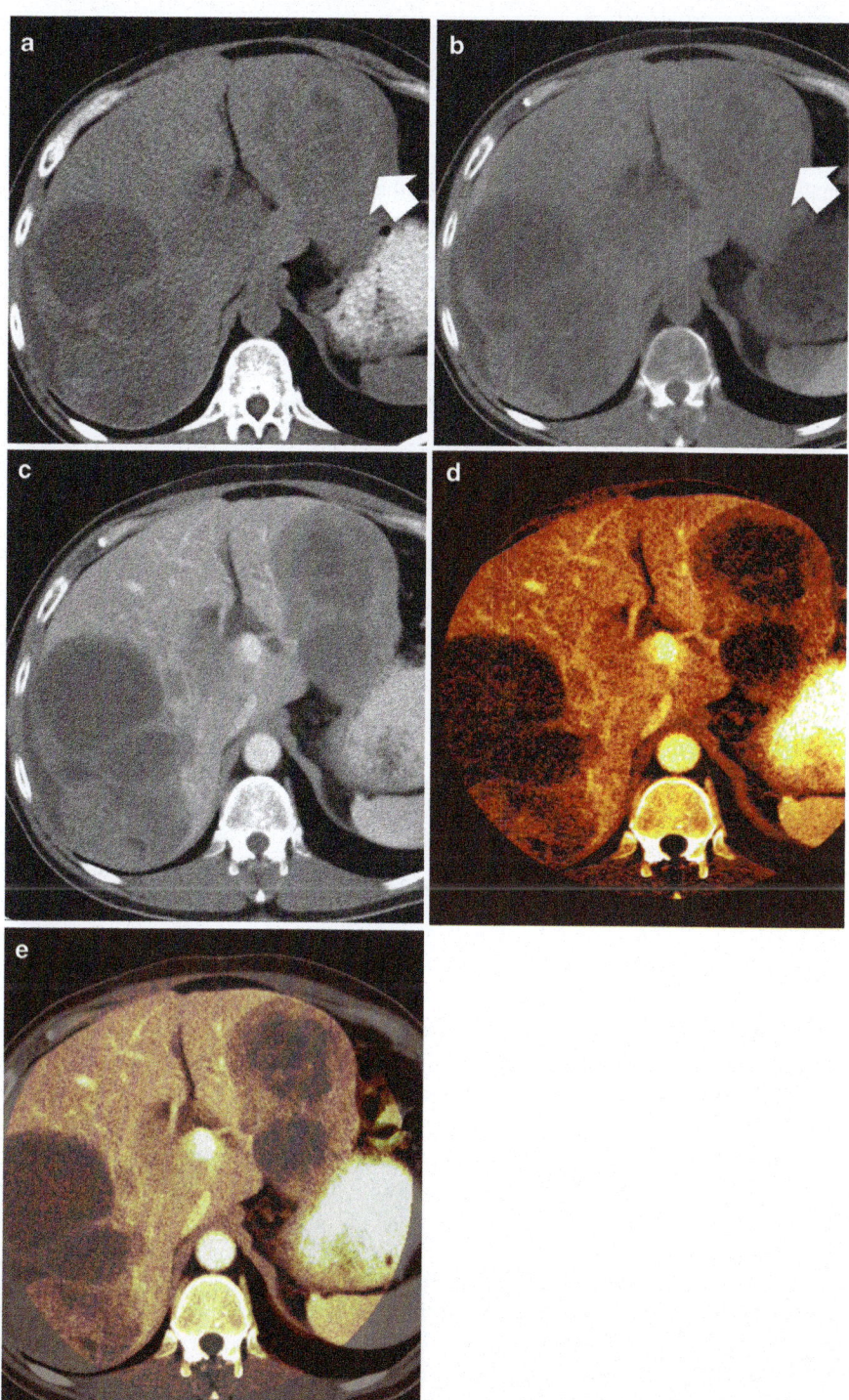

It could be recently demonstrated that DECT is a promising imaging modality for the assessment of treatment response in GIST, as IRA may be a more robust response parameter than Choi criteria [19]. DECT is capable of visualizing and quantifying typical patterns of GIST lesions. Further, DECT analysis is a promising predictor of tumor progression if compared to established response criteria. A recent analysis by Meyer et al. [23] also indicated that DECT allows a better prediction of therapeutic benefit in advanced GIST patients treated with tyrosine kinase inhibitors than established response criteria. However, the most important predictive bio-marker of therapeutic benefit in this study was absence of progression, no matter which response evaluation criteria were applied.

7.3   Duodenal Carcinoma and Other Tumors of the Small Intestine

Small bowel neoplasms, such as adenocarcinoma, carcinoid tumor, lymphoma, or gastro-intestinal stromal tumors, represent a small percentage of gastrointestinal cancers, how-ever do have poor prognosis compared with other gastrointestinal malignancies [33].

Adenocarcinoma is the most common primary malignancy of the small bowel and accounts for 40 % of cancers with predominant location in the duodenum and proxi-mal jejunum, with the incidence decreasing distally [33, 34]. In general, adenocarci-nomas are more frequently found in the jejunum rather than in the ileum, except in patients with Crohn disease who are at higher risk for this specific tumor [35–37].

Carcinoid is the second most common malignancy, accounting for approximately 20–25 % of all small bowel lesions. Carcinoid tumors are more common in the ileum than in the jejunum or duodenum, and lesions may be multiple and/or meta-static at the time of diagnosis [33].

The third and fourth most common neoplasms are non-Hodgkin lymphoma (NHL) and GIST, respectively. NHL is more common in patients with celiac disease and in patients with acquired immune deficiency syndrome (AIDS), and particu-larly prevalent in developing countries [33].

Malignant neoplasms of the mesenteric small bowel are rare conditions, which are often discovered at an evolved stage, resulting in a poor prognosis. Consequently, early detection of small bowel neoplasms is desirable but still challenging unless appropriate imaging methods and protocols are used [35]. CT and MRI imaging have a well-known potential for providing comprehensive information, including intraluminal, mural, and extraintestinal evaluation. The association of CT scanning with luminal distension of the small bowel and intravenous administration of iodin-ated contrast material is the basic concept behind two specific techniques, namely, CT enteroclysis and CT enterography [35, 38, 39]. Briefly, CT enteroclysis, which is based on direct infusion of enteral contrast agent into the mesenteric small bowel through a naso-jejunal tube, provides optimal luminal distension. By contrast, com-puted tomography enterography is based on oral administration of enteral contrast agent [35]. MR enteroclysis is an emerging technique for the evaluation of the mes-enteric small bowel, which provides excellent image quality and sufficient disten-tion of the entire mesenteric small bowel.

On standard CT images acquired at 120 kVp, it might be difficult to discriminate between physiological and abnormal enhancement of the small bowel wall. However, as low kVp images display greater density of contrast agent than standard images, DECT might help to determine the presence of subtle inflammation when data are viewed at 80 kVp [1]. Similarly, in patients with suspected small bowel ischemia, the low 80 kVp images may aid in visual assessment of small bowel enhancement and hence perfusion [1].

Malignant neoplasms of the mesenteric small bowel are rare conditions, which are often discovered at an evolved stage, resulting in a poor prognosis. DECT might help in the task of early detection of small bowel neoplasms; however, this needs to be further evaluated by outcome-based, unbiased, and well-designed prospective studies.

7.4 Colorectal Cancer

Colorectal cancer remains a major cause of morbidity and mortality worldwide, with approximately 609,000 deaths per annum [40]. Survival of patients with colorectal cancer depends primarily on disease stage. The 5-year relative survival rate is 90 % for localized cancers but only 12–19 % for cancers with distant metastases [41, 42]. Traditionally, colorectal cancers have been classified by clinicopathological features, including tumor location, TNM stage, differentiation, and grade. However, this may not provide sufficient information with respect to tumor profiling toward a more targeted treatment approach. Colorectal cancers are heterogeneous with respect to genetic and epigenetic mutations and may be classified by molecular characteristics [40, 43, 44].

Imaging plays an important role in the assessment of colorectal cancer, including diagnosis, staging, selection of treatment, assessment of treatment response, surveillance, and investigation of suspected disease relapse [40]. Concurrent with advances in the treatment of colorectal cancers, there have been major advances in imaging, with the development of new imaging modalities, functional imaging techniques, and contrast media and the proposal of alternative tumor response criteria [42, 45, 46]. Utilization of different imaging modalities in diagnosing of colorectal cancer varies between countries and institutions. Recent developments in imaging technologies and validation of newer imaging techniques may lead to significant improvements in the management of patients with colorectal cancers. Diagnostic techniques such as diffusion-weighted imaging (DWI), fluorodeoxyglucose positron emission tomography (FDG-PET), and dynamic contrast-enhanced magnetic resonance imaging (DCE-MRI) are increasingly used and have shown to be clinically useful in tumor characterization [47–50]. Newly developed techniques such as perfusion CT and MRI spectroscopy allowing insights in tumor biology have shown promising results; however, they are not yet validated for clinical practice [7, 8]. Recently, DECT has been investigated for direct visualization of iodine uptake within tumor in color-coded fashion, which makes a reliable quantification of enhancement [51] (Fig. 7.3). Using redcolor-encoding iodine overlay images generated by DECT, Chen et al. were able to demonstrate the extra colonic spread of the tumor [51]. The fact that cancers show enhancement of approximately 40 HU on

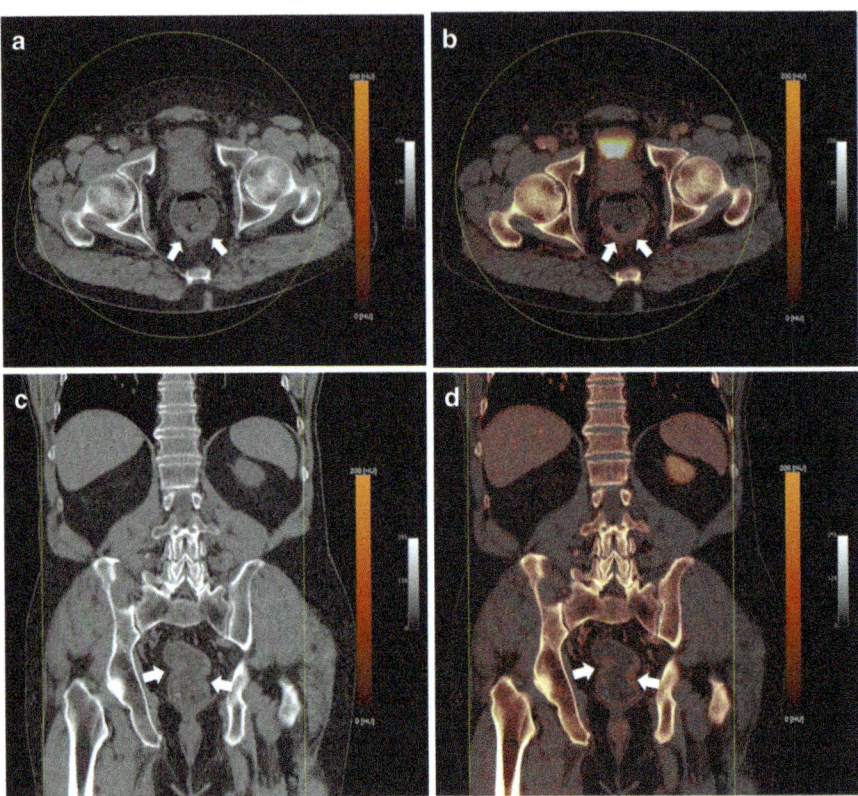

Fig. 7.3 A 67-year-old male with biopsy-proven adenocarcinoma of the rectum shown on axial and coronal non-contrast-enhanced CT images (**a, c**) and axial and coronal fused color-coded iodine maps (**b, d**) (*arrows*). DECT iodine images help differentiate simple nonenhancing heterogeneity, shows excellent delineation of the mass (*arrows*), and provides information on increased iodine uptake of the tumor

single-energy CT during the portal phase strengthens the idea that enhancement of colorectal cancers may be used for their detection, especially when conspicuity can be increased [52–54]. In a feasibility study, Boellaard et al. could show that colorectal cancers are visible on the contrast-enhanced DECT without bowel preparation or insufflation [52]. Because of the patient-friendly nature of this approach, further studies should explore its use for colorectal cancer detection in frail and elderly patients. As technological improvements in CT continue to evolve, this will further extend clinical applications.

Conclusion

DECT is an innovative imaging technique that can have a considerable effect on the care of oncologic patients. The possibility of obtaining different material-specific datasets in oncology has considerable potential for improving tumor detection and characterization while concurrently shortening the examination time and reducing the radiation dose [1, 2, 31, 32]. Additionally, imaging-based therapy monitoring has gained a central role in oncologic imaging and a DECT-based therapy monitoring concept may allow for objective, easy, and fast evaluation of the tumor size and contrast-medium uptake in one step and may have a promising role in monitoring therapy response [2]. Various whole-body applications are conceivable for routine oncological monitoring; however, studies investigating DECT for the gastrointestinal tract are rare, as until recently, the main two focuses for abdominal oncological imaging using DECT were the detection and characterization of focal liver lesions and second oncological imaging of pancreatic cancer. Recent studies suggest that DECT has the potential to improve the differentiation between benign and malignant tissue in gastrointestinal cancers, but more prospective clinical studies are warranted to assess the clinical benefit.

References

1. Graser A, Johnson TR, Chandarana H, Macari M (2009) Dual energy CT: preliminary observations and potential clinical applications in the abdomen. Eur Radiol 19:13–23
2. Simons D, Kachelriess M, Schlemmer HP (2014) Recent developments of dual-energy CT in oncology. Eur Radiol 24:930–939
3. De Cecco CN, Darnell A, Rengo M et al (2012) Dual-energy CT: oncologic applications. AJR Am J Roentgenol 199:S98–S105
4. Fuentes-Orrego JM, Pinho D, Kulkarni NM, Agrawal M, Ghoshhajra BB, Sahani DV (2014) New and evolving concepts in CT for abdominal vascular imaging. Radiographics 34: 1363–1384
5. Agrawal MD, Pinho DF, Kulkarni NM, Hahn PF, Guimaraes AR, Sahani DV (2014) Oncologic applications of dual-energy CT in the abdomen. Radiographics 34:589–612
6. Rosenbaum SJ, Stergar H, Antoch G, Veit P, Bockisch A, Kuhl H (2006) Staging and follow-up of gastrointestinal tumors with PET/CT. Abdom Imaging 31:25–35
7. Levine MSHR (2000) Esophageal carcinoma. Saunders, Philadelphia
8. Wong R, Walker-Dilks C, Raifu A (2012) Evidence-based guideline recommendations on the use of positron emission tomography imaging in oesophageal cancer. Clin Oncol 24:86–104
9. Allum WH, Blazeby JM, Griffin SM, Cunningham D, Jankowski JA, Wong R (2011) Guidelines for the management of oesophageal and gastric cancer. Gut 60:1449–1472
10. van Rossum PS, van Lier AL, Lips IM et al (2015) Imaging of oesophageal cancer with FDG-PET/CT and MRI. Clin Radiol 70(1):81–95
11. Lauren P (1965) The two histological main types of gastric carcinoma: diffuse and so-called intestinal-type carcinoma. An attempt at a histo-clinical classification. Acta Pathol Microbiol Scand 64:31–49
12. Hallinan JT, Venkatesh SK (2013) Gastric carcinoma: imaging diagnosis, staging and assessment of treatment response. Cancer Imaging 13:212–227
13. Cuenod CA, Fournier L, Balvay D, Guinebretiere JM (2006) Tumor angiogenesis: pathophysiology and implications for contrast-enhanced MRI and CT assessment. Abdom Imaging 31:188–193
14. Lee TY, Purdie TG, Stewart E (2003) CT imaging of angiogenesis. Q J Nucl Med 47: 171–187
15. Yao J, Yang ZG, Chen TW, Li Y, Yang L (2010) Perfusion changes in gastric adenocarcinoma: evaluation with 64-section MDCT. Abdom Imaging 35:195–202
16. Miettinen M, Lasota J (2001) Gastrointestinal stromal tumors – definition, clinical, histological, immunohistochemical, and molecular genetic features and differential diagnosis. Virchows Arch 438:1–12

17. Ghanem N, Altehoefer C, Furtwangler A et al (2003) Computed tomography in gastrointestinal stromal tumors. Eur Radiol 13:1669–1678
18. Sureka B, Mittal MK, Mittal A, Sinha M, Thukral BB (2014) Imaging spectrum of gastrointestinal stromal tumor. Indian J Med Paediatr Oncol 35:143–148
19. Apfaltrer P, Meyer M, Meier C et al (2012) Contrast-Enhanced Dual-Energy CT of Gastrointestinal Stromal Tumors: Is Iodine-Related Attenuation a Potential Indicator of Tumor Response? Invest Radiol 47(1)):65–70
20. Demetri GD, Benjamin RS, Blanke CD et al (2007) NCCN Task Force report: management of patients with gastrointestinal stromal tumor (GIST) – update of the NCCN clinical practice guidelines. J Natl Compr Canc Netw 5(Suppl 2):S1–S29, quiz S30
21. Demetri GD, von Mehren M, Blanke CD et al (2002) Efficacy and safety of imatinib mesylate in advanced gastrointestinal stromal tumors. N Engl J Med 347:472–480
22. Benjamin RS, Choi H, Macapinlac HA et al (2007) We should desist using RECIST, at least in GIST. J Clin Oncol 25:1760–1764
23. Meyer M, Hohenberger P, Apfaltrer P et al (2013) CT-based response assessment of advanced gastrointestinal stromal tumor: dual energy CT provides a more predictive imaging biomarker of clinical benefit than RECIST or Choi criteria. Eur J Radiol 82:923–928
24. Choi H (2008) Response evaluation of gastrointestinal stromal tumors. Oncologist 13 (Suppl 2):4–7
25. Choi H, Charnsangavej C, de Castro Faria S et al (2004) CT evaluation of the response of gastrointestinal stromal tumors after imatinib mesylate treatment: a quantitative analysis correlated with FDG PET findings. AJR Am J Roentgenol 183:1619–1628
26. Choi H, Charnsangavej C, Faria SC et al (2007) Correlation of computed tomography and positron emission tomography in patients with metastatic gastrointestinal stromal tumor treated at a single institution with imatinib mesylate: proposal of new computed tomography response criteria. J Clin Oncol 25:1753–1759
27. Hong X, Choi H, Loyer EM, Benjamin RS, Trent JC, Charnsangavej C (2006) Gastrointestinal stromal tumor: role of CT in diagnosis and in response evaluation and surveillance after treatment with imatinib. Radiographics 26:481–495
28. Reichardt P, Schneider U, Stroszczynski C, Pink D, Hohenberger P (2004) Molecular response of gastrointestinal stromal tumour after treatment with tyrosine kinase inhibitor imatinib mesylate. J Clin Pathol 57:215–217
29. Tawfik AM, Kerl JM, Bauer RW et al (2012) Dual-energy CT of head and neck cancer: average weighting of low- and high-voltage acquisitions to improve lesion delineation and image quality-initial clinical experience. Invest Radiol 47:306–311
30. Sommer CM, Schwarzwaelder CB, Stiller W et al (2012) Iodine removal in intravenous dual-energy CT-cholangiography: is virtual non-enhanced imaging effective to replace true non-enhanced imaging? Eur J Radiol 81(4):692–699
31. Neville AM, Gupta RT, Miller CM, Merkle EM, Paulson EK, Boll DT (2011) Detection of renal lesion enhancement with dual-energy multidetector CT. Radiology 259(1):173–183
32. Graser A, Johnson TR, Hecht EM et al (2009) Dual-energy CT in patients suspected of having renal masses: can virtual nonenhanced images replace true nonenhanced images? Radiology 252:433–440
33. Anzidei M, Napoli A, Zini C, Kirchin MA, Catalano C, Passariello R (2011) Malignant tumours of the small intestine: a review of histopathology, multidetector CT and MRI aspects. Br J Radiol 84:677–690
34. Ouriel K, Adams JT (1984) Adenocarcinoma of the small intestine. Am J Surg 147:66–71
35. Soyer P, Boudiaf M, Fishman EK et al (2011) Imaging of malignant neoplasms of the mesenteric small bowel: new trends and perspectives. Crit Rev Oncol Hematol 80:10–30
36. Fidler JL, Guimaraes L, Einstein DM (2009) MR imaging of the small bowel. Radiographics 29:1811–1825
37. Verma D, Stroehlein JR (2006) Adenocarcinoma of the small bowel: a 60-yr perspective derived from M.D Anderson cancer center tumor registry. Am J Gastroenterol 101:1647–1654

38. Maglinte DD, Sandrasegaran K, Lappas JC, Chiorean M (2007) CT enteroclysis. Radiology 245:661–671
39. Romano S, De Lutio E, Rollandi GA, Romano L, Grassi R, Maglinte DD (2005) Multidetector computed tomography enteroclysis (MDCT-E) with neutral enteral and IV contrast enhancement in tumor detection. Eur Radiol 15:1178–1183
40. Goh V, Glynne-Jones R (2014) Perfusion CT imaging of colorectal cancer. Br J Radiol 87:20130811
41. Kopetz S, Chang GJ, Overman MJ et al (2009) Improved survival in metastatic colorectal cancer is associated with adoption of hepatic resection and improved chemotherapy. J Clin Oncol 27:3677–3683
42. Tirumani SH, Kim KW, Nishino M et al (2014) Update on the role of imaging in management of metastatic colorectal cancer. Radiographics 34:1908–1928
43. Vogelstein B, Fearon ER, Hamilton SR et al (1988) Genetic alterations during colorectal-tumor development. N Engl J Med 319:525–532
44. Shen L, Toyota M, Kondo Y et al (2007) Integrated genetic and epigenetic analysis identifies three different subclasses of colon cancer. Proc Natl Acad Sci U S A 104:18654–18659
45. Fowler KJ, Linehan DC, Menias CO (2013) Colorectal liver metastases: state of the art imaging. Ann Surg Oncol 20:1185–1193
46. Chun YS, Vauthey JN, Boonsirikamchai P et al (2009) Association of computed tomography morphologic criteria with pathologic response and survival in patients treated with bevacizumab for colorectal liver metastases. JAMA 302:2338–2344
47. Kekelidze M, D'Errico L, Pansini M, Tyndall A, Hohmann J (2013) Colorectal cancer: current imaging methods and future perspectives for the diagnosis, staging and therapeutic response evaluation. World J Gastroenterol 19:8502–8514
48. Torigian DA, Huang SS, Houseni M, Alavi A (2007) Functional imaging of cancer with emphasis on molecular techniques. CA Cancer J Clin 57:206–224
49. Beets-Tan RG, Beets GL, Vliegen RF et al (2001) Accuracy of magnetic resonance imaging in prediction of tumour-free resection margin in rectal cancer surgery. Lancet 357:497–504
50. Niekel MC, Bipat S, Stoker J (2010) Diagnostic imaging of colorectal liver metastases with CT, MR imaging, FDG PET, and/or FDG PET/CT: a meta-analysis of prospective studies including patients who have not previously undergone treatment. Radiology 257:674–684
51. Chen CY, Hsu JS, Jaw TS et al (2014) Utility of the iodine overlay technique and virtual non-enhanced images for the preoperative T staging of colorectal cancer by dual-energy CT with tin filter technology. PLoS One 9, e113589
52. Boellaard TN, Henneman OD, Streekstra GJ et al (2013) The feasibility of colorectal cancer detection using dual-energy computed tomography with iodine mapping. Clin Radiol 68:799–806
53. Neri E, Vagli P, Picchietti S et al (2005) CT colonography: contrast enhancement of benign and malignant colorectal lesions versus fecal residuals. Abdom Imaging 30:694–697
54. Oto A, Gelebek V, Oguz BS et al (2003) CT attenuation of colorectal polypoid lesions: evaluation of contrast enhancement in CT colonography. Eur Radiol 13:1657–1663

Dual Energy CT in Renal Tumors

8

Achille Mileto and Daniele Marin

8.1 Introduction

The advent of multidetector row CT (MDCT) in the early 2000s has dramatically changed the imaging approach to genitourinary disease, especially renal masses imaging. By exploiting the increased coverage along the z-axis and taking full advantage of the rapid image acquisition, genitourinary *MDCT* protocols relies on scanning the kidney and urinary tract with a multiphasic approach, before and after contrast medium administration [1–3].

With the expanding use of MDCT, the number of *renal lesions* that is incidentally discovered has increased. While a definite diagnosis can be confidently posed for most of them, a number of renal lesions remain indeterminate following MDCT examinations [1–6]. Under such circumstances, further imaging tests are typically prescribed, ensuing in an increase of healthcare costs, radiation exposure, and patient's anxiety.

By addressing most of the drawbacks of conventional MDCT imaging, *dual energy MDCT* can improve the diagnosis of renal lesions and, potentially, may represent a paradigm shift from a merely attenuation-based to a material-specific spectral imaging investigation. In this chapter, we provide an overview of currently available clinical applications of dual energy MDCT in the evaluation of renal lesions.

8.2 Renal Lesions: From Conventional to Dual Energy MDCT

Multi-detector row computed tomography (MDCT) has become the optimal imaging modality for characterizing and staging renal lesions [1–3]. Routine MDCT imaging protocols for renal lesion characterization include an unenhanced

A. Mileto • D. Marin (✉)
Department of Radiology, Duke University Medical Center,
DUMC Box 3808, Durham, NC 27710, USA
e-mail: achille.mileto@duke.edu; daniele.marin@duke.edu

© Springer International Publishing Switzerland 2015
C.N. De Cecco et al. (eds.), *Dual Energy CT in Oncology*,
DOI 10.1007/978-3-319-19563-6_8

followed by contrast-enhanced acquisitions acquired at one to three different time points after the injection of contrast material, including corticomedullary, nephrographic, and excretory phases of enhancement (approximately 40 s, 90 s, and 8 min after injection of contrast agent, respectively) [1–6]. The nephrographic phase should always be acquired [1–6] and represents the ideal time point for identifying and, along with the unenhanced phase, for characterizing renal lesions based on the evaluation of lesion enhancement [2–5]. Corticomedullary and excretory phases are often acquired to provide additional valuable information for the presurgical planning and assessment of the collecting system anatomy [2–6]. Nevertheless, an important consideration to this multiphase technique is the high radiation exposure to patients [1–6].

As the use of MDCT expanded, an increasing number of *renal lesions* were serendipitously discovered. While the majority of them represent benign *renal cysts*, not all incidental renal lesions are benign [1–5, 7, 8]. Up to 61 % of renal cell carcinomas (RCCs) are asymptomatic and are discovered incidentally during abdominal CT performed for other clinical indications [9]. Therefore, differentiating incidental benign renal lesions from those that are potentially malignant is an important and common clinical task [1–5, 7–11]. Nonetheless, this task is frequently challenged by a variety of technical factors inherent to a conventional MDCT technique. These include an inadequate acquisition protocol (most commonly the absence of unenhanced images), potential spatial misregistration due to multiphase examinations as well as equivocal levels of renal lesions contrast-enhancement (attenuation increase, 10–20 HU) [12–15].

Dual energy MDCT enables novel and unique applications to address some of the challenges associated with *conventional MDCT* techniques and has the potential to dramatically change the clinical approach to renal lesions imaging [16–33]. The possibility of substantially reducing radiation dose exposure by decreasing the number of imaging phases (with virtual unenhanced images reconstruction and subsequent omission of standard unenhanced acquisition) in genitourinary protocols has represented the initial clinical application of dual energy MDCT in imaging *renal lesions* [18–27]. The detection and quantification of materials allow the radiologist to calculate lesion iodine uptake in single-phase nephrographic images [14, 26, 34]. Further, recent developments in dual energy technology permit to synthesize virtual monochromatic images by applying a spectral separation to polychromatic source data. This has the potential to provide more accurate and more reproducible attenuation measurements [35–37].

8.3   Dual Energy MDCT Applications for Renal Lesions Imaging

Dual energy MDCT applications employed for imaging renal masses can be categorized into methods for displaying "energy-specific" data or providing "material-specific" information. While "energy-specific" techniques rely on providing MDCT quantitative information in Hounsfield units (HU), "material-specific" applications also allow for providing the radiologist with direct measures of material densities (in mg/mL).

8.3.1 Energy-Specific Applications

8.3.1.1 Technical Considerations

On the basis of material decomposition and the knowledge of mass attenuation of materials, *dual energy MDCT* enables the creation of *virtual monochromatic images* by applying a mathematic model to the source polychromatic data obtained from acquiring data with two energy spectra [35, 36, 38]. Depending on the MDCT system used to acquire the dual energy data, the approach to base material decomposition slightly differs. Notably, for dual energy MDCT data acquired with a single-source fast kV switching technique, the base material decomposition is performed in the data domain. By comparison, for dual energy MDCT data acquired with a dual-source MDCT system, material decomposition analysis is performed in the image domain. This is primarily because the projection data from the low- and high-energy projections collected by the dual-source system in helical mode are not coincident with each other [35–39]. For a given photon energy, virtual monochromatic images (whose energy is reported as keV instead of kV) mimic those images that would result from a true monochromatic x-ray source [35–39]. The advantage of a monochromatic beam is that it is less susceptible to beam-hardening phenomena and therefore has the potential to provide more accurate and more reproducible *attenuation measurements* over those obtained with a conventional MDCT technique [35–39].

8.3.1.2 Clinical Applications

Preliminary data demonstrated that virtual monochromatic datasets can overcome renal cyst pseudoenhancement within an energy level range of 80–140 keV (Fig. 8.1) [38]. This yields an unequivocal diagnosis of simple *renal cysts*, eliminating the need of additional work-up [37].

By exploiting a real-time interactive display of monochromatic images at a dual energy workstation, the radiologist can interrogate the change in attenuation of a lesion over a range of discrete energies, a process that is not feasible with *conventional MDCT* [35, 36]. In particular, with the use of dedicated software applications, keV spectral attenuation curves can be generated by plotting the attenuation values (in HU) of a material at different monochromatic energies, ranging from 40–140 keV. With this technique, specific tissue characterization is achievable based on known mean attenuation characteristics of different materials, especially those with higher atomic numbers [35, 36]. Enhancing solid *renal lesions* can be potentially differentiated from nonenhancing cysts on a single-phase nephrographic image based on spectral attenuation curves. Of note, solid tumors uptaking iodine show a steep increase in

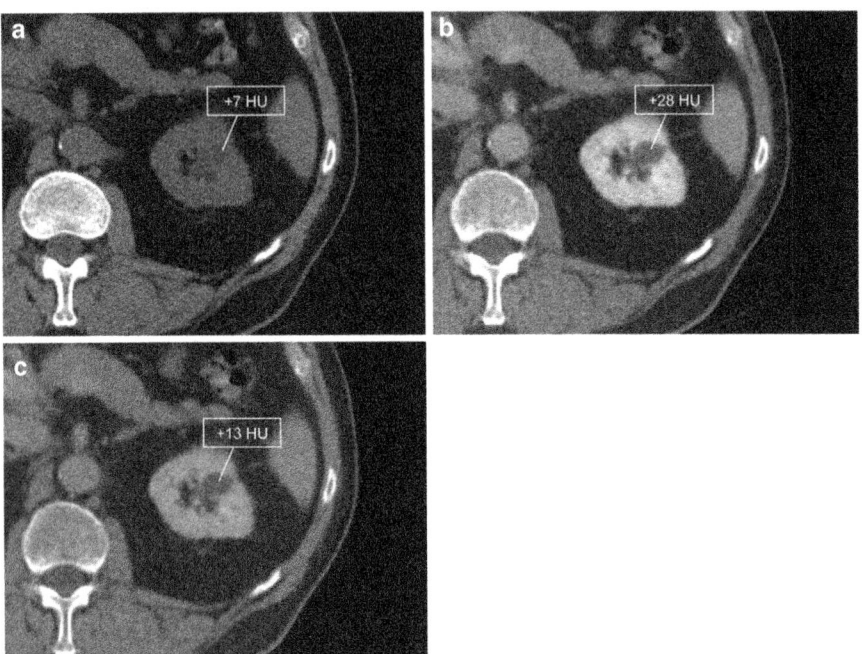

Fig. 8.1 (**a**) Conventional noncontrast, postcontrast, (**b**) conventional, and (**c**) 80 keV virtual monochromatic nephrographic images in a 45-year-old man with low attenuation intra-parenchymal lesion of the left kidney. In the unavailability of a (**a**) conventional noncontrast scan, the lesion is called indeterminate on the basis of (**b**) conventional postcontrast nephrographic imaging. The (**c**) 80 keV virtual monochromatic nephrographic image allows for minimizing pseudoenhancement, hence warranting a definite diagnosis of simple cyst

attenuation with progressive lower energies (upward curve), whereas nonenhancing cysts do not modify their attenuation across the explored monochromatic scale (flat curve) (Figs. 8.2 and 8.3).

8.3.2 Material-Specific Applications

8.3.2.1 Technical Considerations

Material-specific images can be obtained from dual energy data, either after the reconstruction of high- and low-energy images ("image-domain decomposition") or before images are reconstructed from high- and low-energy sinograms ("data-domain" or "projection-space decomposition") [23, 35–43]. Image-domain decomposition is used for material analysis of images obtained with the dual-source MDCT system, whereas data-domain decomposition is used for material analysis of *dual energy MDCT* images obtained with fast kV switching MDCT platform [23, 35–43].

Information from dual energy datasets allow for the analysis of material composition in a voxel-by-voxel fashion based on either a "three-material-decomposition"

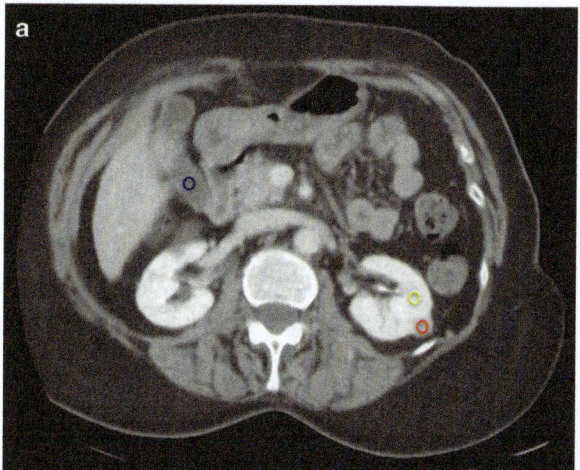

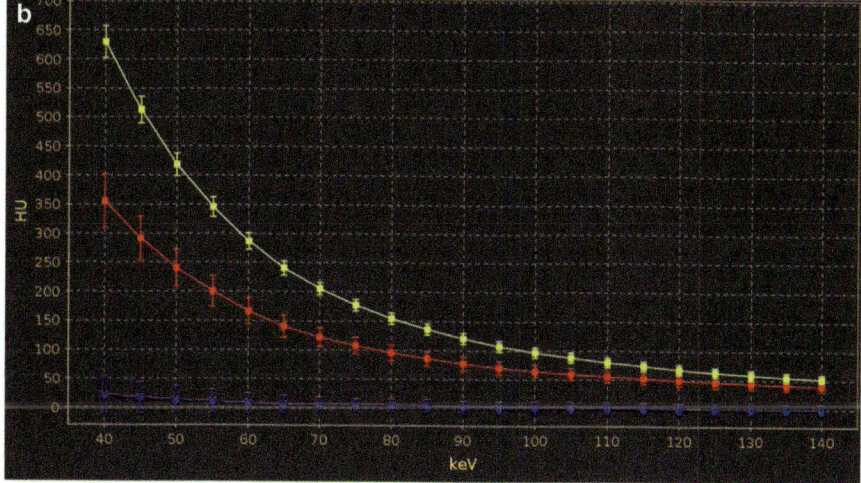

Fig. 8.2 (**a**) Contrast-enhanced 70 keV virtual monochromatic nephrographic phase transverse image with (**b**) corresponding spectral attenuation curve calculation in a 64-year-old man with high-attenuation lesion of the left kidney. There is possible concern of lesion enhancement; however, in the absence of unenhanced imaging, a certain diagnosis cannot be made as the lesion may represent either an enhancing lesion or a high-attenuation cyst. (**b**) ROIs are placed on the renal lesion (*red* ROI), normal renal parenchyma (*yellow* ROI) and within the gallbladder (*azure* ROI). By plotting the attenuation values of a material at different monochromatic energies, ranging from 40 to 140 keV, the corresponding spectral attenuation curve is generated for the three ROIs at various keV values. The renal lesion shows a relatively steep, upwardly sloping curve (*red curve*) at lower keV, which resembles that of enhancing normal renal parenchyma (*yellow curve*) while substantially differing from that of the nonenhancing gallbladder fluid (*azure curve*), The analysis of these spectral curves allows one for concluding that the renal lesion represents an enhancing solid tumor

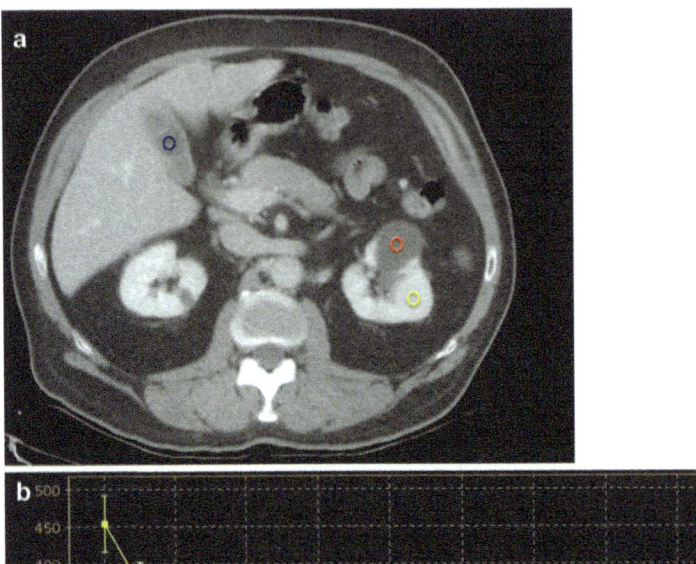

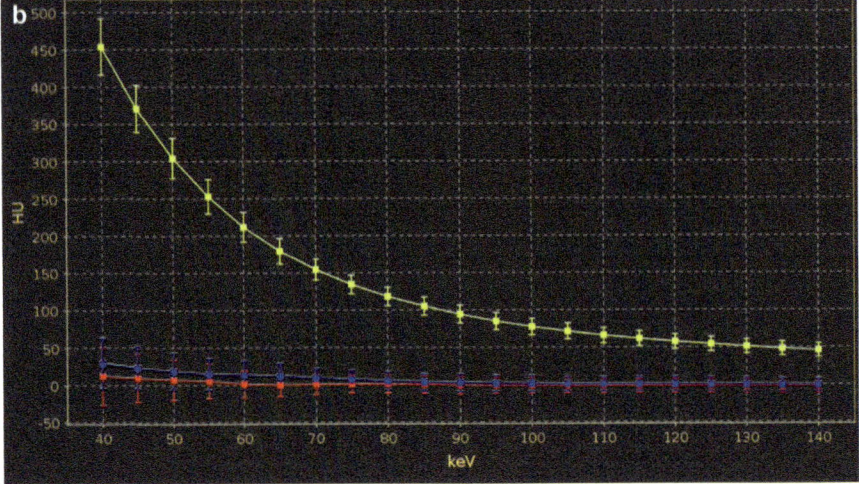

Fig. 8.3 (**a**) Contrast-enhanced 70 keV virtual monochromatic nephrographic phase transverse image with (**b**) spectral attenuation curve calculation in a 57-year-old man with low-attenuation lesion of the left kidney. (**b**) ROIs are placed on the renal lesion (*red* ROI), normal renal parenchyma (*yellow* ROI) and within the gallbladder (*azure* ROI). By plotting the attenuation values of a material at different monochromatic energies, ranging from 40 to 140 keV, the corresponding spectral attenuation curve is generated for the three ROIs at various keV values. The renal lesion shows a flat curve (*red curve*) at lower keV, which resembles that of the nonenhancing gallbladder fluid (*azure curve*), while substantially differing from that of enhancing normal renal parenchyma (*yellow curve*). The analysis of these spectral curves allows one for concluding that the renal lesion represents a nonenhancing cyst

principle for image domain decomposition or a "two-material-decomposition" principle for data-domain decomposition [23, 35–43]. With a three-material-decomposition analysis, the absorption characteristics of three idealized materials, such as fat, soft tissue, and iodine, are used at two energy levels to create a spectral

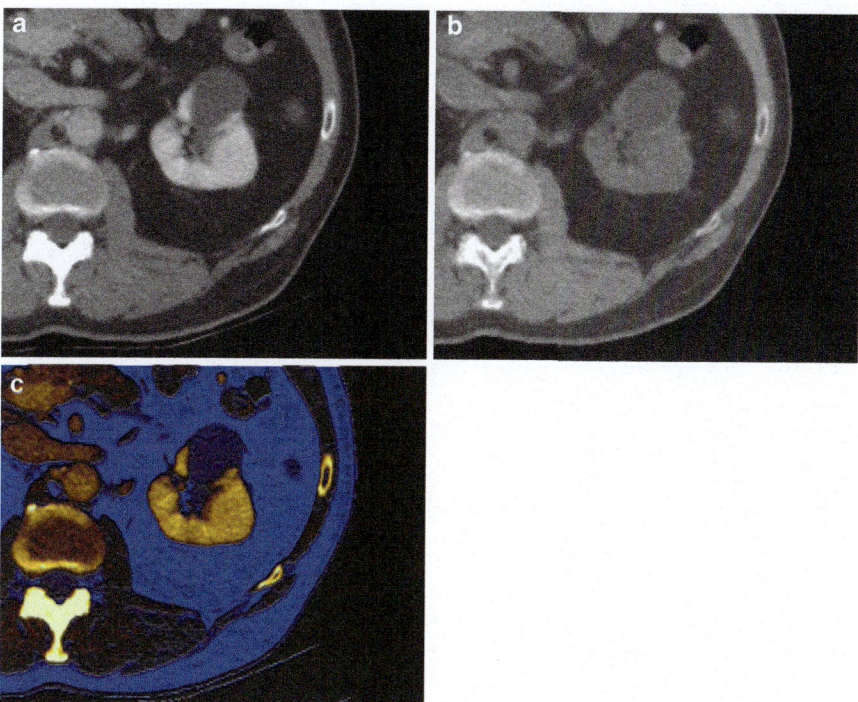

Fig. 8.4 Dual energy material decomposition analysis, including (**a**) conventional nephrographic, (**b**) virtual unenhanced, and (**c**) color-coded iodine map, in a 57-year-old man with a nonenhancing cystic lesion of the left kidney. Note that enhancement, by means of color signal devoid, is confidently ruled out in the lesion on the (**c**) color-coded iodine map

iodine extraction image series; the iodine contribution to the image can be subtracted, thus generating a virtual unenhanced images or, alternatively, can be overlaid in different percentages on gray-scale information, thus creating a color-coded *iodine map* [23, 35–43]. By comparison, when a two-material decomposition algorithm is utilized, the absorption characteristics of two basis materials (i.e., iodine and calcium, or iodine and water) having substantially different effective atomic number and mass-attenuation coefficients are used to obtain two sets of images ("material-density images") [23, 35–43]. Specifically, if iodine and water are the selected base materials, iodine- and water-density images are obtained (Figs. 8.4 and 8.5).

8.3.2.2 Clinical Applications

Along with baseline attenuation measurements, the evaluation of lesion morphologic and structural features represents a critical step in the characterization of a renal mass [1–9, 19]. Of note, when a *renal lesion* shows enhancement in the concurrent presence of intralesional calcifications, and possibly macroscopic fat, it should be considered suspicious for malignancy [1–9, 19]. *Virtual unenhanced images* have demonstrated to be quantitatively and qualitatively comparable to conventional unenhanced images

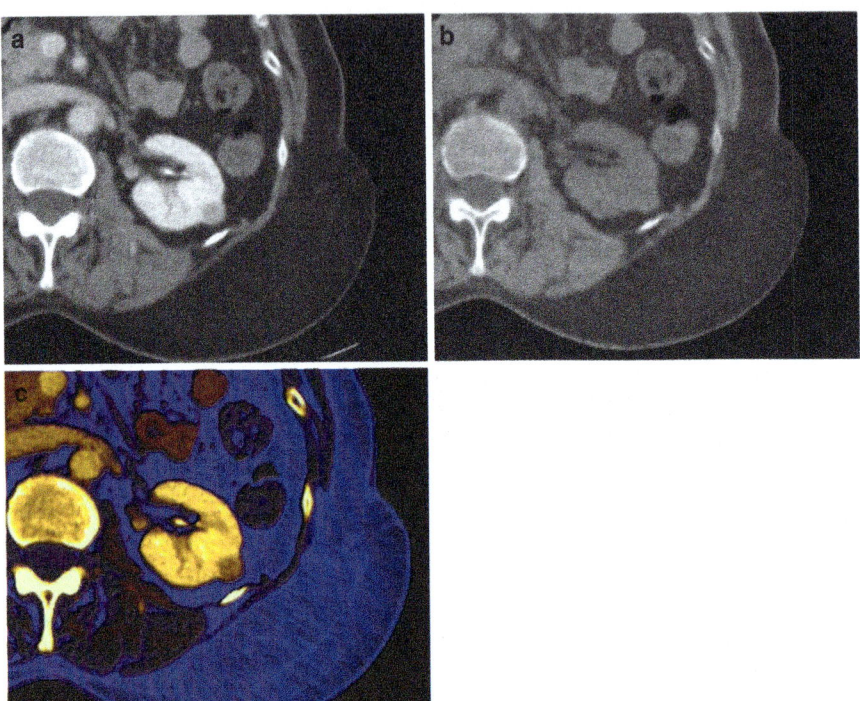

Fig. 8.5 Dual energy material decomposition analysis, including (**a**) conventional nephrographic, (**b**) virtual unenhanced, and (**c**) color-coded iodine map, in a 64-year-old man with renal cell carcinoma of the left kidney. Note that enhancement, by means of color signal, is confidently identified in the lesion on the (**c**) color-coded iodine map

[14, 16–19, 21–23, 25, 28, 31, 32]. An accumulating body of evidence in literature has shown that virtual unenhanced images represent a clinically feasible surrogate of conventional noncontrast images for various anatomic regions throughout the abdomen and, specifically, allow for reliable assessment of pre-contrast renal lesion attenuation [14, 16–19, 21–23, 25, 28, 31, 32]. Furthermore, virtual unenhanced images are able to depict a broad range of different structural features that may be found in a renal lesion, including areas of low attenuation (e.g., fat, cystic components, or necrosis), intermediate attenuation (e.g., solid component or debris), high attenuation (e.g., hemorrhagic or protein-rich content), as well as calcifications [16, 19, 21–23, 25, 28, 31, 32]. Thereby, virtual unenhanced imaging allows for omitting the acquisition of conventional noncontrast images, translating into achieving in daily clinical practice a 30 % mean dose saving for triphasic and up to 50 % for biphasic renal MDCT protocols. This may be particularly beneficial to decrease the cumulative radiation dose in patients requiring long-term *MDCT* follow-up (i.e., young patients with complex cystic renal lesions) [14–17, 19, 22, 23, 25].

A daily question oftentimes the radiologist is faced in clinical practice is the differential diagnosis between benign high-attenuation cysts (Bosniak category II) and solid enhancing lesions (most importantly renal cell carcinoma) on contrast-enhanced images, if the measured attenuation of a renal lesion is higher than the attenuation of simple fluid (>+20 HU). High-attenuation cysts (due to hemorrhagic or protein-rich content) are homogeneous, well-defined lesions without evidence of enhancement [1–9, 19–49]. The latter is the diagnostic clue for differentiating a high-attenuation cyst from an enhancing solid *renal neoplasm*, especially when an enhancing renal mass is small, well-defined, and homogeneous in attenuation. Under these circumstances, if a noncontrast acquisition is not available, the patient must undergo either: (a) an ultrasound (which is often not definitive, especially if the attenuation of the lesion is greater than +40 HU because it contains blood or proteinaceous debris), (b) an additional delayed CT acquisition to assess for "de-enhancement" or, more commonly, (c) a repeated study with either *MDCT* or MRI which includes both unenhanced and contrast-enhanced acquisitions [49]. Iodine-specific dual-energy images (color-coded iodine overlay or iodine-density images) allows for a color-coded display of the iodine distribution within the explored volume [17–23, 25–28, 30, 36–39, 47, 50]. The direct visualization of iodine signal within the mass permit to distinguish a nonenhancing cyst from a solid enhancing lesion on a single-phase color-coded iodine image. Of note, as *renal cysts* are avascular, color-coded iodine-specific images show a cyst as devoid of iodine signal (Fig. 8.4). By comparison, enhancing solid renal masses demonstrate iodine signal within the lesion (Fig. 8.5) [17–23, 25–28, 30, 36–39, 47].

Color-coded iodine overlay images can also provide further benefits over conventional MDCT imaging for the evaluation of enhancement in subcentimeter renal masses. This subset is usually prone to substantial variability in region-of-interest (ROI) placement, especially on renal tumors that are isodense to the renal parenchyma on noncontrast images [1–9, 15, 26, 39, 42, 43]. As the presence of enhancement within a renal lesion can be determined without the need for MDCT number measurements on both unenhanced and contrast-enhanced images, one can refrain from unenhanced images acquisition and postprocessing (Fig. 8.6) [19, 22, 26, 28]. It has been demonstrated that renal lesions can be accurately characterized in a single-phase dual energy protocol, with image interpretation time and radiation exposure that are significantly decreased [14, 19, 22, 25, 26, 28].

More recently, *dual energy MDCT* also enables a direct quantification of iodine concentration (in mg/mL) in a lesion with a single ROI on color-coded iodine images [14, 26, 34]. This represents an alternative approach to conventional attenuation measurements for the determination of lesion enhancement, relying on the assumption that iodine does not naturally occur in measurable concentrations in the healthy renal tissue; the only way it can be present is through exogenous administration [14, 26, 34]. A burgeoning evidence in literature has been suggesting that iodine quantification may be superior to conventional attenuation measurements, especially in discriminating minimally enhancing tumors, such as papillary subtypes of renal cancer, from high-attenuation cysts [14, 26, 34]. Of note, a lesion iodine

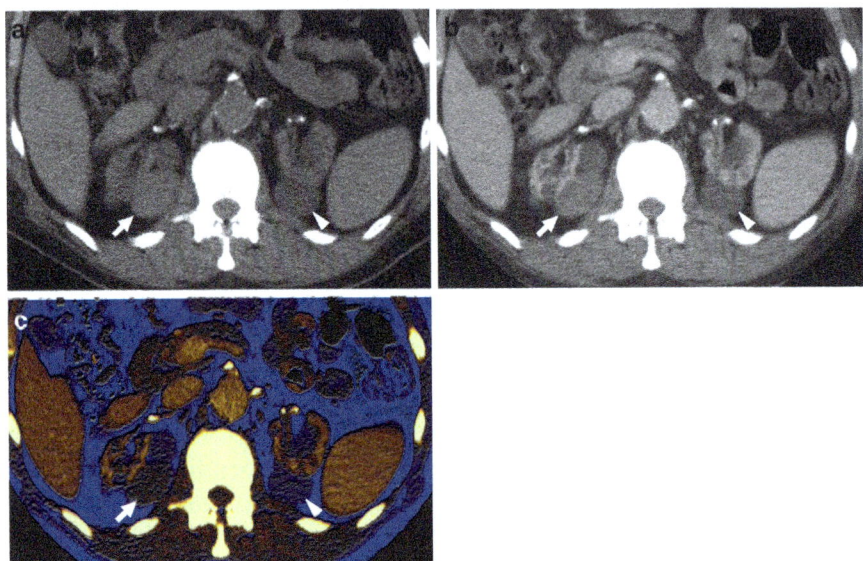

Fig. 8.6 (**a**) Conventional noncontrast, postcontrast, (**b**) conventional nephrographic, and (**c**) color-coded iodine map images are shown in a 65-year-old man with multiple, bilateral renal lesions. There is possible concern of lesions enhancement, especially for two lesions arising from the medial aspect of the right (*arrow*) and the left (*arrowhead*) kidney. The use of (**c**) color-coded iodine map allows for confidently identifying iodine content (1.4 mg/mL) within the lesion (RCC) located in the right kidney (*arrow*), while ruling out any enhancement in the lesion of the left kidney (*arrowhead*)

concentration greater than 0.5 mg/mL has been suggested as highly indicative of renal lesion iodine uptake (Fig. 8.6) [14, 26].

While large ROIs are typically adopted for ascertaining the presence of enhancement in *renal lesions* showing homogeneous texture, multiple small ROI measurements, which have to be obtained from all portions of the lesion and similarly placed on both the unenhanced and contrast-enhanced images, are required for complex cystic or necrotic lesions [2–6]. This approach is often tedious, depends on reader's experience, and is affected by the inclusion of small areas of necrosis or cystic changes. While conventional enhancement measurements are affected by the inclusion of necrosis or cystic areas because it is the averaged value of all areas within the ROI, the iodine concentration is the summed value of enhancing areas alone and thus this value is not affected by the inclusion of necrosis or cystic areas within the ROI [26]. Therefore, independent of the solid or cystic tumor texture, it is possible to accurately assess the iodine uptake by drawing a single large ROI on color-coded iodine image [14, 26]. This allows elimination of all confounding factors in *enhancement* evaluation and to significantly reduce reading time.

Another clinical scenario where color-coded iodine overlay images may be of clinical use is the imaging surveillance after percutaneous thermal ablation of a renal mass. In such a clinical context, *conventional MDCT* imaging is used periodically to assess the effectiveness of the treatment and to determine the presence of complications, such as tumor recurrence [51–54]. Of note, the presence of tissue

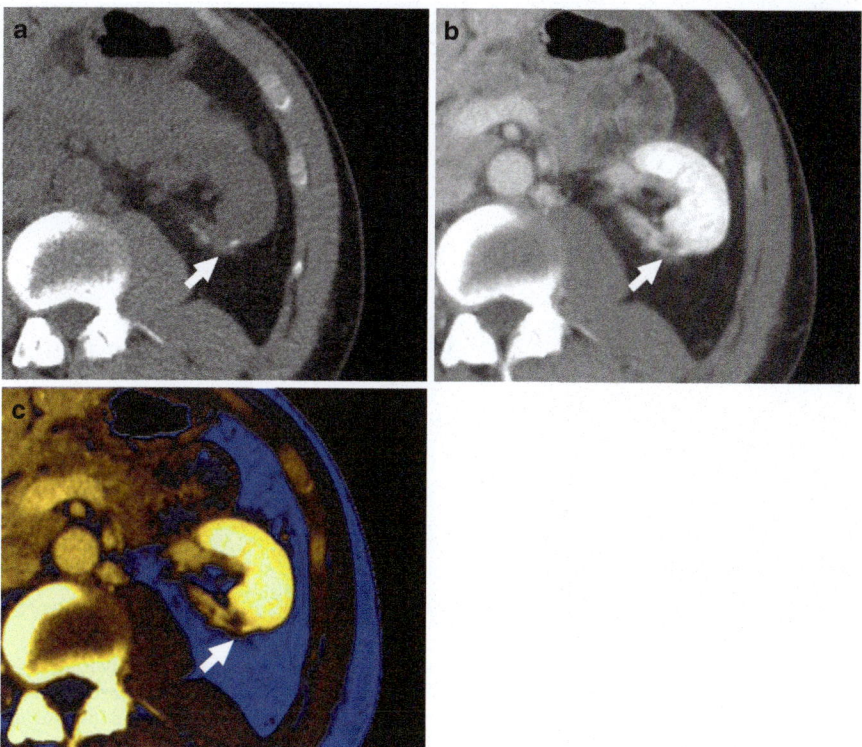

Fig. 8.7 (**a**) Conventional noncontrast, postcontrast, (**b**) conventional nephrographic, and (**c**) color-coded iodine map images are shown in a 61-year-old man who underwent cryoablation of an RCC of the left kidney. On postcontrast (**b**) conventional nephrographic images, there is concern of enhancement in the cryoablation bed (*arrow*), which could not be excluded in the potential unavailability of (**a**) conventional noncontrast images. By selective display of iodine-containing voxels, color-coded iodine map (**c**) image permits one to clearly rule out any tumor recurrence within the ablation site, as a devoid of signal is seen (*arrow*)

enhancement and nodular growth are the two imaging features commonly used to identify remaining viable tissue after ablation of a *renal tumor* [51–54]. Nevertheless, changes due to the prior ablation treatment, such as perinephric hematoma and stranding, can complicate the identification of tumor recurrence at MDCT [51–54]. By virtue of the selective representation of iodine-containing voxels, *dual energy MDCT* iodine density and color-coded iodine overlay images may represent a problem-solving tool in this clinical context (Fig. 8.7).

8.4   Pitfalls

A number of potential *pitfalls* has, however, to be cautiously considered when *dual energy MDCT* is adopted for imaging the renal mass.

Owing to the inherent limitations of the employed algorithms used to discriminate among materials having similar attenuation coefficient energy dependencies (e.g., iodine,

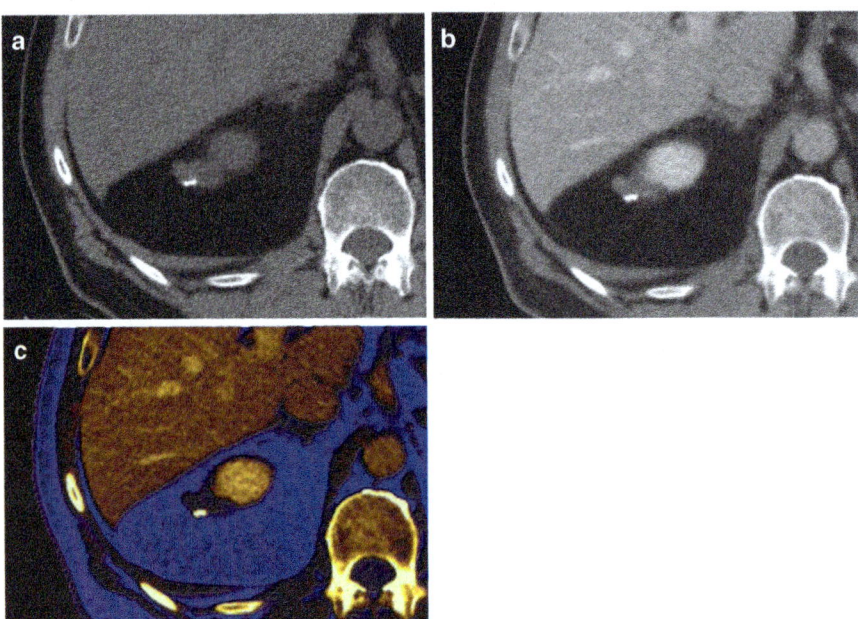

Fig. 8.8 (**a**) Conventional noncontrast, postcontrast, (**b**) conventional nephrographic, and (**c**) color-coded iodine map images are shown in a 58-year-old man with a Bosniak category II complicated cyst of the right kidney. A calcified septation is identified on conventional (**a, b**) imaging. Note the spurious signal within the septation seen on the (**c**) iodine map

iron, and calcium), it oftentimes happens that lesions containing either high concentration of hemoglobin or coarse calcification may be misinterpreted as displaying iodine content on iodine maps (Fig. 8.8) [16, 21, 22]. On the other hand, the inability to distinguish between iodine and either calcium or iron in a renal mass using this technique could make the characterization of *RCC* challenging at times [16, 21, 22].

Although robust data supports the clinical use of virtual unenhanced datasets as a method of containing the radiation dose burden to patients [16, 21, 22], an incomplete subtraction of iodine contrast can oftentimes occur, especially with some of the early dual energy scanners (i.e., due to limited separation of the two energy spectra) as well as in the presence of extremely high iodine concentrations (e.g., during peak of nephrographic parenchymal enhancement) [16, 21, 22].

Despite the theoretical monochromatic nature, currently available virtual monochromatic datasets at suggested optimal energy levels (e.g., 80–140 keV for overcoming renal cyst pseudoenhancement) can suffer from residual beam-hardening effects especially in large patients [35, 37]. This implies that in this patient subset, higher monochromatic energy levels (≥90 keV) should be selected in order to fully correct for renal cyst pseudoenhancement [35, 37].

Finally, as for other abdominal clinical settings, an appropriate patient selection may be of critical importance when dual energy MDCT is performed on a routine daily basis. Specifically, it has been shown that beyond certain patient body sizes (e.g., greater than 250 lb), the increased noise and beam-hardening artifacts occurring with the low energy data make the dual energy scan mode highly inadvisable because substantial image quality degradation may occur for all reconstructed dual energy datasets [55].

8.5   Future Perspectives

Future perspectives for *dual energy MDCT renal lesions* imaging may be opened up by the implementation of iodine-specific dual energy imaging differentiating between different subtypes of *RCC*, determining the tumor grade, and assessing the response to targeted therapy in metastatic RCC [14]. The adoption of iodine quantification as imaging biomarker of tumor viability may provide additional information over CT numbers in the depiction of tumor texture heterogeneity in RCC as well as in demonstrating early changes to therapy that go beyond macroscopic tumor shrinkage [14, 26]. Additional applications may be derived from the calculation of effective atomic numbers and dual energy indexes from density maps [35, 36, 39].

Conclusions

Dual energy MDCT provides radiologists with a promising, powerful technology that has the potential to improve the imaging-based diagnosis and, potentially, the management of *renal masses*, while the radiation dose exposure to patients is substantially decreased.

In the near future, dual energy MDCT may enable paradigm shift for renal lesions CT imaging, from a merely attenuation-based to a material-specific spectral imaging investigation in which iodine, due to its physical properties, can be used as a "biological tracer" of *iodine uptake*.

References

1. Kang SK, Chandarana H (2012) Contemporary imaging of the renal mass. Urol Clin North Am 39:161–170
2. Israel GM, Silverman SG (2011) The incidental renal mass. Radiol Clin North Am 49:369–383
3. Israel GM, Silverman SG (2008) Management of the incidental renal mass. Radiology 249:16–31
4. Israel GM, Bosniak MA (2008) Pitfalls in renal mass evaluation and how to avoid them. Radiographics 28:1325–1338
5. Israel GM, Bosniak MA (2005) How I do it: evaluating renal masses. Radiology 236:441–450
6. Birnbaum BA, Jacobs JE, Ramchandani P (1996) Multiphasic renal CT: comparison of renal mass enhancement during the corticomedullary and nephrographic phases. Radiology 200:753–758
7. Decastro GJ, McKiernan JM (2008) Epidemiology, clinical staging, and presentation of renal cell carcinoma. Urol Clin North Am 35:581–592
8. Neville AM, Gupta RJ, Miller CM, Merkle EM, Paulson EK, Boll DT (2011) Detection of renal lesion enhancement with dual-energy multidetector CT. Radiology 259:173–183

9. Suh M, Coakley FV, Qayyum A, Yeh BM, Breiman SB, Lu Y (2003) Distinction of renal cell carcinomas from high-attenuation renal cysts at portal venous phase contrast-enhanced CT. Radiology 228:330–334

10. Goyal A, Sharma R, Bhalla AS, Gamanagatti S, Seth A (2013) Diffusion-weighted MRI in inflammatory renal lesions: all that glitters is not RCC! Eur Radiol 23:272–279

11. Karlo CA, Donati OF, Burger IA et al (2013) MR imaging of renal cortical tumours: qualitative and quantitative chemical shift imaging parameters. Eur Radiol 23(6):1738–1744

12. Birnbaum BA, Hindman N, Lee J et al (2007) Multidetector row CT attenuation measurements: assessment of intra- and interscanner variability with an anthropomorphic body CT phantom. Radiology 242:109–119

13. Birnbaum BA, Hindman N, Lee J et al (2007) Renal cyst pseudoenhancement: influence of multidetector CT reconstruction algorithm and scanner type in phantom model. Radiology 244:767–775

14. Chandarana H, Megibow AJ, Cohen BA et al (2011) Iodine quantification with dual energy CT: phantom study and preliminary experience with renal masses. AJR Am J Roentgenol 196:W693–W700

15. Jinzaki M, McTavish JD, Zou KH, Judy PF, Silverman SG (2004) Evaluation of small (≤3 cm) renal masses with MDCT: benefits of thin overlapping reconstructions. AJR Am J Roentgenol 183:1223–1228

16. Graser A, Johnson TR, Hecht EM et al (2009) Dual energy CT in patients suspected of having renal masses: can virtual nonenhanced images replace true nonenhanced images? Radiology 252:433–440

17. Graser A, Johnson TR, Chandarana H, Macari M (2009) Dual energy CT: preliminary observations and potential clinical applications in the abdomen. Eur Radiol 19:13–23

18. Johnson TR, Krauss B, Sedlmair M et al (2007) Material differentiation by dual energy CT: initial experience. Eur Radiol 17:1510–1517

19. Ascenti G, Mazziotti S, Mileto A et al (2012) Dual-source dual energy CT evaluation of complex cystic renal masses. AJR Am J Roentgenol 199:1026–1034

20. Brown CL, Hartman RP, Dzyubak OP et al (2009) Dual energy CT iodine overlay technique for characterisation of renal masses as cyst or solid: a phantom feasibility study. Eur Radiol 19:1289–1295

21. Fletcher JG, Takahashi N, Hartman R et al (2009) Dual-energy and dual-source CT: is there a role in the abdomen and pelvis? Radiol Clin North Am 47:41–57

22. Graser A, Becker CR, Staehler M et al (2010) Single-phase dual energy CT allows for characterisation of renal masses as benign or malignant. Invest Radiol 45:399–405

23. Kaza R, Caoili EM, Cohan RH, Platt JF (2011) Distinguishing enhancing from nonenhancing renal lesions with fast kilovoltage-switching dual energy CT. AJR Am J Roentgenol 197:1375–1381

24. Ascenti G, Krauss B, Mazziotti S et al (2012) Dual-energy computed tomography (DECT) in renal masses: nonlinear versus linear blending. Acad Radiol 19:1186–1193

25. Ascenti G, Mileto A, Gaeta M, Blandino A, Mazziotti S, Scribano E (2013) Single-phase dual energy CT urography in the evaluation of haematuria. Clin Radiol 68:87–94

26. Ascenti G, Mileto A, Krauss B et al (2013) Distinguishing enhancing from nonenhancing renal masses with dual-source dual energy CT: iodine quantification versus standard enhancement measurements. Eur Radiol 23(8):2288–2295

27. Song KD, Kim CK, Park BK, Kim B (2011) Utility of iodine overlay technique and virtual unenhanced images for the characterisation of renal masses by dual energy CT. AJR Am J Roentgenol 197:1076–1082

28. Arndt N, Staehler M, Siegert S, Reiser MF, Graser A (2012) Dual energy CT in patients with polycystic kidney disease. Eur Radiol 22:2125–2129

29. Miller CM, Gupta RT, Paulson EK et al (2011) Effect of organ enhancement and habitus on estimation of unenhanced attenuation at contrast-enhanced dual-energy MDCT: concepts for individualized and organ-specific spectral iodine subtraction strategies. AJR Am J Roentgenol 196:W558–W564

30. Karlo C, Lauber A, Götti RP et al (2011) Dual energy CT with tin filter technology for the discrimination of renal lesion proxies containing blood, protein, and contrast-agent. An experimental phantom study. Eur Radiol 21:385–392

31. Mileto A, Mazziotti S, Gaeta M et al (2012) Pancreatic dual-source dual energy CT: is it time to discard unenhanced imaging? Clin Radiol 67:334–339

32. Ascenti G, Mazziotti S, Lamberto S et al (2011) Dual energy CT for detection of endoleaks after endovascular abdominal aneurysm repair: usefulness of coloured iodine overlay. AJR Am J Roentgenol 196:1408–1414

33. Petersilka M, Bruder H, Krauss B, Stierstorfer K, Flohr TG (2008) Technical principles of dual source CT. Eur J Radiol 68:362–368

34. Feuerlein S, Heye TJ, Bashir MR, Boll DT (2012) Iodine quantification using dual-energy multidetector computed tomography imaging: phantom study assessing the impact of iterative reconstruction schemes and patient habitus on accuracy. Invest Radiol 47:656–661

35. Yu L, Leng S, McCollough CH (2012) Dual energy CT–based monochromatic imaging. AJR Am J Roentgenol 199:S9–S15

36. Silva AC, Morse BG, Hara AK, Paden RG, Hongo N, Pavlicek W (2011) Dual-energy (spectral) CT: applications in abdominal imaging. Radiographics 31:1031–1046

37. Mileto A, Nelson RC, Samei E et al (2014) Impact of dual-energy multi-detector row CT with virtual monochromatic imaging on renal cyst pseudoenhancement: in vitro and in vivo study. Radiology 272:767–776

38. Fornaro J, Leschka S, Hibbeln D et al (2012) Dual- and multi-energy CT: approach to functional imaging. Insights Imaging 2:149–159

39. Hartman R, Kawashima A, Takahashi N et al (2012) Applications of dual energy CT in urologic imaging: an update. Radiol Clin North Am 50:191–205

40. Qu M, Jaramillo-Alvarez G, Ramirez-Giraldo JC et al (2013) Urinary stone differentiation in patients with large body size using dual-energy dual-source computed tomography. Eur Radiol 23(5):1408–1414

41. Apel A, Fletcher JG, Fidler JL et al (2011) Pilot multi-reader study demonstrating potential for dose reduction in dual energy hepatic CT using non-linear blending of mixed kV image data-sets. Eur Radiol 21:644–652

42. Kaza RK, Platt JF, Megibow AJ (2013) Dual energy CT of the urinary tract. Abdom Imaging 38:167–179

43. Kaza RK, Platt JF, Cohan RH, Caoili EM, Al-Hawary MM, Wasnik A (2012) Dual energy CT with single- and dual-source scanners: current applications in evaluating the genitourinary tract. Radiographics 32:353–369

44. Boll DT, Patil NA, Paulson EK et al (2009) Renal stone assessment with dual-energy multidetector CT and advanced postprocessing techniques: improved characterisation of renal stone composition—pilot study. Radiology 250:813–820

45. Boll DT, Merkle EM, Paulson EK, Mirza RA, Fleiter TR (2008) Calcified vascular plaque specimens: assessment with cardiac dual-energy multidetector CT in anthropomorphically moving heart phantom. Radiology 249:119–126

46. Coursey CA, Nelson RC, Boll DT et al (2010) Dual-energy multidetector CT: how does it work, what can it tell us, and when can we use it in abdominopelvic imaging? Radiographics 30:1037–1055

47. Heye T, Nelson RC, Ho LM, Marin D, Boll DT (2012) Dual energy CT applications in the abdomen. AJR Am J Roentgenol 199:S64–S70

48. Boll DT, Patil NA, Paulson EK et al (2010) Focal cystic high-attenuation lesions: characterisation in renal phantom by using photon-counting spectral CT-improved differentiation of lesion composition. Radiology 254:270–276

49. Macari M, Bosniak MA (1999) Delayed CT to evaluate renal masses incidentally discovered at contrast-enhanced CT: demonstration of vascularity with deenhancement. Radiology 213:674–680

50. Leschka S, Stolzmann P, Baumüller S et al (2010) Performance of dual-energy CT with tin filter technology for the discrimination of renal cysts and enhancing masses. Acad Radiol 17:526–534

51. Ljungberg B, Cowan C, Hanbury DC et al (2010) European association of urology guideline group. EAU guidelines on renal cell carcinoma: the 2010 update. Eur Urol 58:398–406
52. Rosenkrantz AB, Sekhar A, Genega EM et al (2013) Prognostic implications of the magnetic resonance imaging appearance in papillary renal cell carcinoma. Eur Radiol 23:579–587
53. Solomon SB, Silverman SG (2010) Imaging in interventional oncology. Radiology 257: 624–640
54. Kawamoto S, Permpongkosol S, Bluemke DA, Fishman EK, Solomon SB (2007) Sequential changes after radiofrequency ablation and cryoablation of renal neoplasms: role of CT and MR imaging. Radiographics 27:343–355
55. Guimarães LS, Fletcher JG, Harmsen WS et al (2010) Appropriate patient selection at abdominal dual-energy CT using 80 kV: relationship between patient size, image noise, and image quality. Radiology 257:732–742

Dual Energy CT in Musculoskeletal Tumors

9

Colin Chun Wai Chong, Shamir Rai, and Savvas Nicolaou

Abbreviations

DECT   Dual–energy computed tomography
kV   Kilovoltage
VNC   Virtual noncontrast

9.1 Introduction

All patients suspected of having a primary soft tissue or bone sarcoma at our institution receive comprehensive imaging. Plain radiographs, ultrasounds, and conventional tomography (CT) are usually the initial imaging investigation in assessing "lumps and bumps." Magnetic resonance imaging (MRI) is the most comprehensive modality for assessing tumor extent and has excellent soft tissue contrast resolution [1, 2]. Positron emission tomography (PET) scans can assess for metabolic activity in a lesion and assess treatment response [1, 3–5]. Once the appropriate imaging investigations have been performed, the patients are discussed in a multidisciplinary team meeting comprised of surgical orthopedic oncologists, medical oncologists, radiation oncologists, musculoskeletal radiologists, and pathologists. Subsequently, the majority of these patients undergo pretreatment percutaneous biopsy at our

C.C.W. Chong (✉) • S. Nicolaou
Department of Radiology, Vancouver General Hospital,
855 West 12th Avenue, Vancouver, BC, Canada
e-mail: drcolincwchong@gmail.com

S. Rai
Faculty of Medicine, University of British Columbia,
Vancouver, BC, Canada

© Springer International Publishing Switzerland 2015
C.N. De Cecco et al. (eds.), *Dual Energy CT in Oncology*,
DOI 10.1007/978-3-319-19563-6_9

institution. Imaging plays a key role in developing a management plan and an appropriate approach for biopsy, surgery, chemotherapy, or radiotherapy as required.

There have been significant technological advances in the imaging of bone and soft tissue tumours, particularly with modern CT and MRI scanners. Oncologic orthopedic surgical techniques have also progressed from limb amputation to "limb sparing surgery." This often involves wide surgical margins around the tumor and adjuvant chemotherapy and/or radiotherapy, with the aim of preserving the patient's limb and function [3, 4, 6, 7].

The advent of DECT has resulted in a paradigm shift and reinvigoration of the utilization of CT in musculoskeletal (MSK) imaging. Currently in MSK imaging, DECT is most commonly used in the detection of uric acid deposits in the assessment of gout [6, 8–10]. DECT provides promising clinical applications and enhanced capabilities in oncological imaging, particularly in primary diagnosis. It has been recognized that there are clear advantages of DECT in tumor detection and lesion characterization within the genitourinary, abdominal, and chest body regions [8, 9, 11, 12]. Through the application of two distinct energy settings, it is possible to differentiate various body substances on the basis of material decomposition [11, 13–17]. Differentiation and characterization of materials are based on the principle that substances with high and low molecular weight composition demonstrate different attenuation behaviors at different energy levels [8, 14, 18, 19]. The technique works particularly well for compounds with a large atomic number by taking advantage of the photoelectric effect [11, 14, 17, 18, 20, 21]. The photoelectric effect predominates at the low kV spectrum because the attenuation value increases exponentially based on the principle that the photoelectric effect is nearly proportional to the third power of the atomic number of the compound and inversely proportional to the third power of the energy level used. A dual energy index value can be calculated for each tissue based on the differentiation of attenuation values at the low and high kV spectrum, which is based on the differences in their atomic weight composition [11, 14, 15, 17, 20, 21]. A greater difference in the dual energy index values provides better characterization and differentiation of the materials in question [6, 11, 15, 22].

The data derived from DECT can be manipulated with specialized software on advanced workstations to analyze tissues with different properties. Applications directly relevant to musculoskeletal oncology will be discussed in this chapter.

Musculoskeletal DECT applications are well established for the assessment of gout, bone marrow edema, and the ability to reduce beam-attenuating artifacts secondary to metal prosthesis using monoenergetic functionality [23, 24]. Studies have also assessed the usefulness of DECT in assessing tendons and ligaments with positive results [11, 25].

At our institution, we utilize a 128-slice dual source DECT system (SOMATOM Definition Flash, Siemens Healthcare), which uses two different x-ray sources simultaneously. This eliminates misregistration of data or errors due to patient movement between acquisitions. Both tubes are operated at different voltages, 80 kV or 100 kV, and 140 kV, with a tin filter. The postprocessing software (Syngo Via Dual Energy, Siemens Healthcare) allows the user to obtain additional information about the chemical composition of body tissue. CT images taken simultaneously with two different kV levels from the same patient and of the same anatomical region are utilized. The differences in the energy dependence of the attenuation coefficients of different materials are exploited. Materials behave differently at different energies, depending on the elements of which they are composed [9, 26]. These images are combined and analyzed to visualize information about anatomical and pathological structures. Color-coded cross-sectional images and three-dimensional (3-D) surface-rendered models can be produced and viewed 360° around any axis. In this chapter, we will explore different application classes with different parameters and algorithms that are clinically relevant to the assessment of soft tissue and bone lesions in the musculoskeletal system.

9.2   Clinical Applications in Musculoskeletal Oncology

9.2.1   The Great Mimicker—Gout Application

Gout is a metabolic condition that results from longstanding hyperuricemia, leading to deposition of monosodium urate (MSU) crystals [11]. The gouty urate tophus is a hallmark of chronic gout [6, 26–28]. The tophus consists of nodular or mass-like aggregates of urate crystals that are surrounded by vascularized granulation tissue and inflammatory infiltrate. The gouty tophus is essentially a foreign body granulomatous response to MSU crystals [14, 17]. Tophi can be seen in periarticular subcutaneous tissues, intraarticular space, tendons, ligaments, cartilage, bone, bursae, and other synovial spaces. Intraosseous tophi can present as cysts or focal sclerotic lesions, if calcified [11]. Faint calcification can be present in 50 % of tophi [2, 15, 29].

Gout, often termed the "great mimicker," most frequently presents at the first metatarsophalangeal joint with the second most common site being at the knee [2, 29–32]. However, gout can present anywhere in the musculoskeletal system. Gout is the most common crystal deposition arthropathy and is a common condition within the general population [2, 30–33]. The incidence and prevalence of gout has increased in recent decades [2, 29, 31, 33].

Uncommon manifestations of a common disease, such as gout, occasionally present as a soft tissue mass suspected to be sarcoma or neoplasia. Upadhyah and Saifuddin recently reported 27 cases of gout that were initially referred to their institution as suspected soft tissue sarcoma [2, 29, 34, 35]. Cases of gout mimicking other tumors have also been reported [2, 34–39]. In particular, gout and synovial sarcoma have been reported to mimic each other [2, 36–40]. This is not surprising as these two distinct conditions share key imaging characteristics such as periarticular location (or location close to a tendon or bursa) and calcification [2, 39, 40]. Indolent nonaggressive erosions can be seen in both gout and synovial sarcoma and thus cannot be used as a reliable differentiating imaging feature [7, 39, 40].

Limited evidence in the literature, including a deficiency of validation in large studies, has resulted in lack of consensus regarding the specificity of established signs of chronic gout, including the classic well-defined punched out erosions with overhanging edge [2, 40, 41]. Furthermore, the sensitivity of these radiographic signs has been reported to be low [12, 29, 41]. Upadhyah and Saifuddin have reported tendon involvement as a nonrecognized imaging feature of gout, which is similar to our institution's experience [11, 29, 42].

MRI is considered the gold standard imaging modality for assessing soft tissue masses [8, 15, 19, 42]. Tophi characteristically show homogeneous, low to intermediate signal intensity on T1-weighted images. Signal intensity on T2-weighted images is variable and depends on the degree of hydration of the tophus and its calcium concentration [11, 15, 29, 43]. Gadolinium-enhanced images demonstrate an intense enhancement of tophus due to proliferative hypervascular synovitis and hypervascular granulation tissue surrounding the tophus [15, 29, 43]. However, none of these MRI imaging features is specific for gout. Various conditions that resemble gouty tophi, in terms of MRI signal characteristics, include rheumatoid arthritis, calcium pyrophosphate disease, xanthofibromas, benign fibroblastic tumors, amyloidosis, pigmented villonodular synovitis, synovial osteochondromatosis, hemophilic arthritis, and granulomatous arthritis such as tuberculosis and fungal infections [13, 15, 16]. The role of MRI at our institution is to assess for features of conditions considered in the differential diagnosis such as the presence of hemosiderin, which is considered to be nearly pathognomonic of PVNS [13, 16, 20, 21].

Ultrasound has been reported to be specific for imaging MSU crystal deposits on hyaline cartilage, known as the "double contour sign" [20, 21]. However, this sonographic sign is of little value in the assessment of soft tissue and bony masses. On ultrasound, the gouty tophus has variable echotexture and consists of inhomogeneous material surrounded by a small anechoic rim, with or without posterior acoustic shadowing depending on the presence of calcification. Doppler ultrasound may demonstrate peripheral hyperemia [15, 20, 21]. The sonographic differential diagnosis of gouty tophi is nonspecific and can be observed in other subcutaneous nodules [15, 22]. At our institution, the role of ultrasound in evaluating soft tissue mass is primarily to distinguish between solid and cystic masses and to guide tissue biopsy.

A small study of 4 patients suggested conventional CT could detect MSU crystals as round or ovoid hyperdense opacities [22]. However, conventional CT lacks the ability to reliably distinguish MSU crystals from calcium based on attenuation values [6, 22].

By contrast, DECT has the key advantage in its ability to differentiate MSU crystals from soft tissue and calcific/osseous mineralization [6, 11, 26]. After loading the two different data sets obtained simultaneously on the DECT into the postprocessing software, an image-based three-material decompositional algorithm of the datasets is subsequently performed to separate calcium from monosodium urate, using soft tissue as the baseline. Reliable classification of the chemical composition of scanned tissues is achieved via material-specific differences in attenuation between the high and low tube voltage acquisitions. Calcium, which is a high molecular weight compound ($Z=20$), has significantly higher attenuation values on 80 kVp as compared to 140 kVp due to the photoelectric effect which allows for accurate material decomposition with post process algorithms. Whereas, low atomic number components such as uric acid composed of hydrogen, oxygen, carbon, nitrogen, and sodium ($Z=1$, $Z=8$, $Z=6$, $Z=7$ and $Z=11$) do not have a significantly higher attenuation value on 80 kVp as compared to 140 kVp images [6, 11, 26]. This allows specific separation of MSU from calcium utilizing a color-coded map highlighting the material in question, for instance, highlighting uric acid in green, cortical calcium in blue, and trabecular calcium in pink [6, 27]. DECT provides good diagnostic accuracy for the detection of MSU deposits in patients with gout. The sensitivity and specificity of DECT against a combined reference standard (polarizing and electron microscopy of synovial fluid) for diagnosing gout has been reported as 0.90 (95 % CI 0.76–0.97) and 0.83 (95 % CI 0.68–0.93), respectively [27, 44].

However, only one study has directly compared DECT with gold standard histology [29, 44]. In this study, gouty tophi were obtained from the cadaveric feet of a single patient with tophaceous gout. Histological analysis of gouty tophi was then correlated with DECT. This case report suggests that DECT highlights dense tophi corresponding to approximately 15 – 20 vol% urate in the tophus. This study suggests that DECT detection is strongly influenced by the variable dense packing of the MSU crystals in the central zone of the tophus. CT simulations performed in this study indicate that mixtures of MSU with water with more than 20 % MSU will exceed the detection threshold of the specific gout algorithm used in this study. The detection thresholds drop to 15 % MSU if MSU is embedded in soft tissue and to an even lower concentration if embedded in tendon. More extensive studies assessing the specificity and sensitivity of MSU crystals against the gold standard of histology are required at this time.

Upadhyah and Saifuddin noted that the nonspecific imaging features of soft tissue masses, even those with a differential diagnosis that includes gout, can make it difficult to reassure clinicians, often leading to recommendation for image-guided biopsy [2, 29]. They also alluded to the role of DECT in replacing the need for needle biopsy. At our institution, we recommend DECT assessment, prior to biopsy, for any mass located around a joint, tendon, or bursa when gout is considered in the differential diagnosis. Following consultation with the referring orthopedic oncologist, a biopsy is performed if the DECT is negative for MSU crystals and annulled when MSU crystals are detected. We present four cases from our institution in Figs. 9.1, 9.2, 9.3, 9.4, and 9.5. The differential diagnoses in these cases include bilateral intraosseous distal tibial giant cell tumor (Fig. 9.1), soft tissue sarcoma (Figs. 9.2 and 9.3), giant cell tumor of the tendon sheath (Fig. 9.4), and localized intraarticular form of pigmented villonodular synovitis (Fig. 9.5). We have found DECT to be an efficient, specific, and noninvasive problem-solving tool for differentiating gouty tophi from other benign and malignant soft tissue and bony masses. DECT can prevent unnecessary biopsy, reduce delays in diagnosis, and minimize morbidity resulting from misdiagnosis.

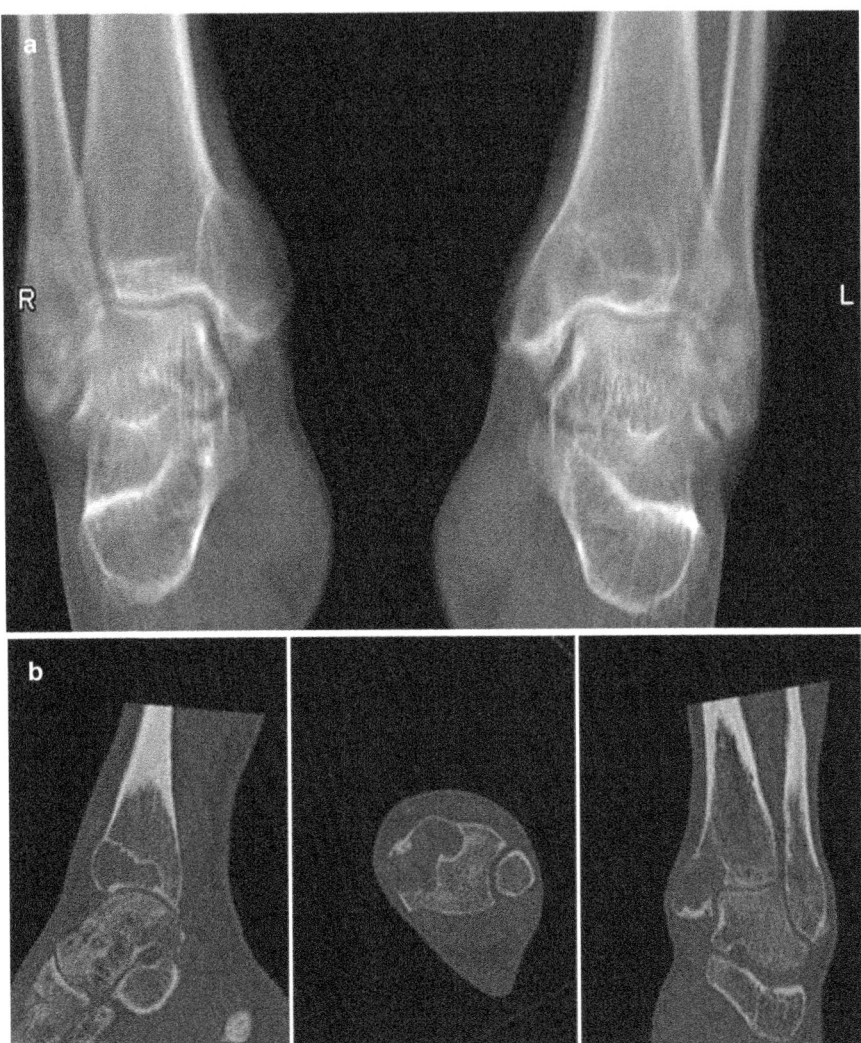

Fig. 9.1 A 56-year old man presented with bilateral medial malleolus acute pain without history of trauma. Erythrocyte sedimentation rate (ESR) was negative. There was no history of gout, malignancy, or infection. Plain radiographs demonstrated intraosseous mass and the patient was subsequently referred to the orthopedic oncology surgeon for work-up and biopsy. Frontal radiographic images (**a**) of bilateral ankles in a patient; (**b**) sagittal, axial, and coronal CT images of the right ankle demonstrate well-marginated lucent lesions in the medial aspect of the distal tibial metaphysis and distal tibial plafond with sclerotic margins. The patient was referred to a sarcoma surgeon for work-up and biopsy. (**c**) coronal STIR, (**d**) coronal T1, and (**e**) axial fat saturated T1 post intravenous gadolinium MR images of the right ankle revealed the mass is hyperintense on STIR and isointense on T1 with predominantly peripheral and mild internal enhancement. (**f**) Bone scan shows increased radiotracer uptake in both these ankle lesions. Coronal (**g**), axial (**h**), and sagittal (**i**) reformatted images from DECT analysis demonstrate monosodium urate deposits within these masses, consistent with intraosseous gout. Uric acid level that was measured after the DECT scan was elevated. No biopsy was performed and the patient was treated conservatively

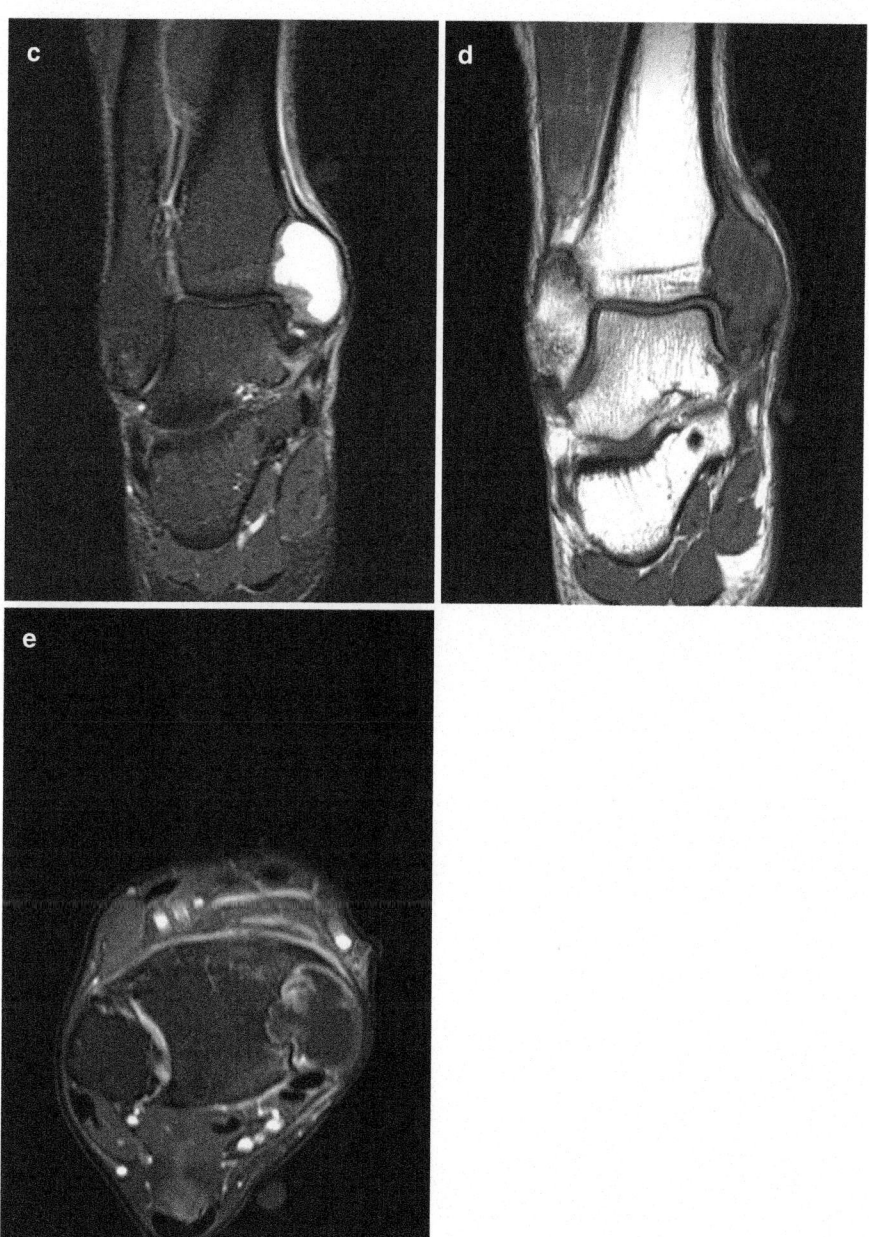

Fig. 9.1 (continued)

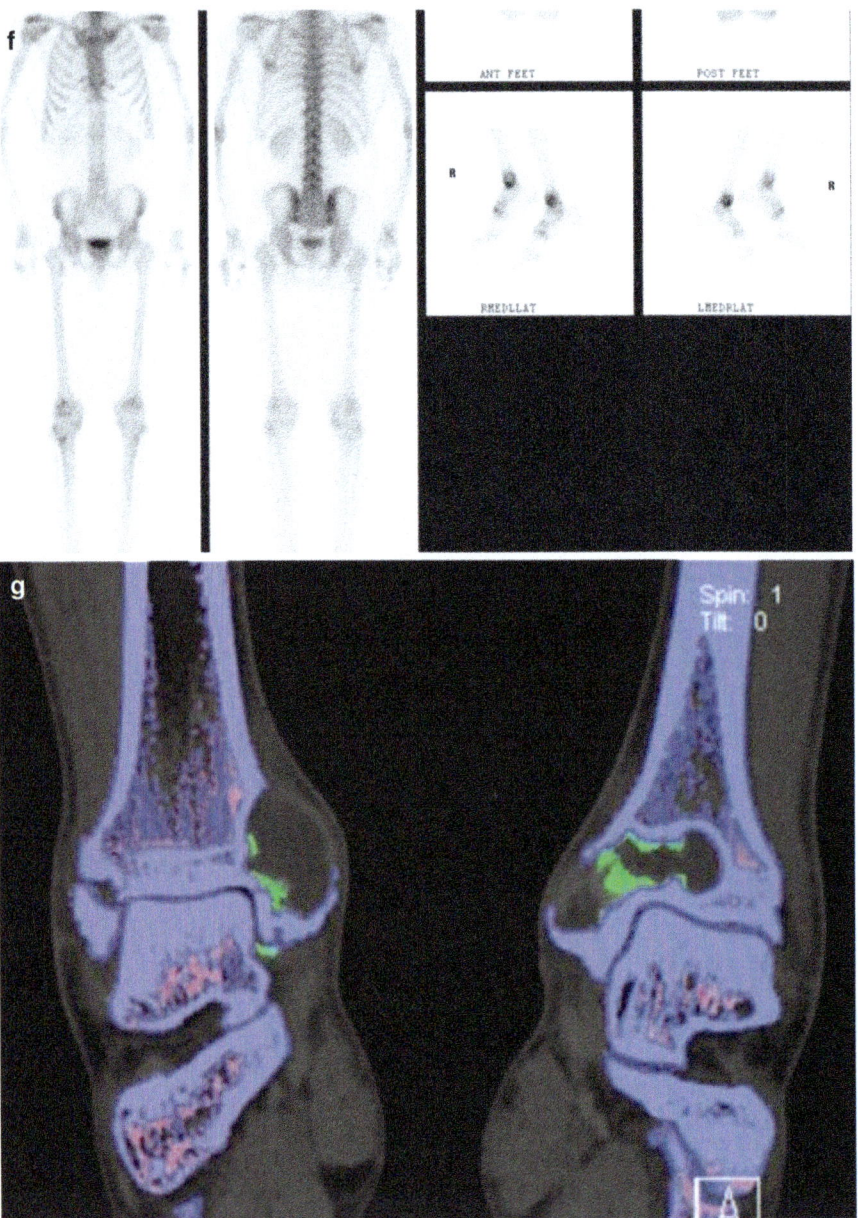

Fig. 9.1 (continued)

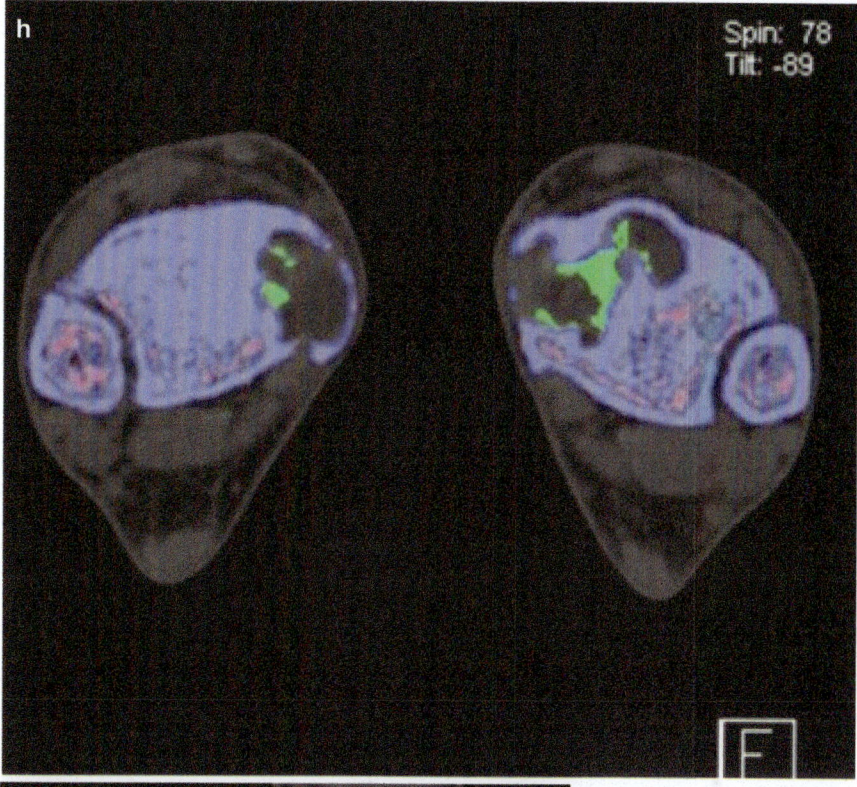

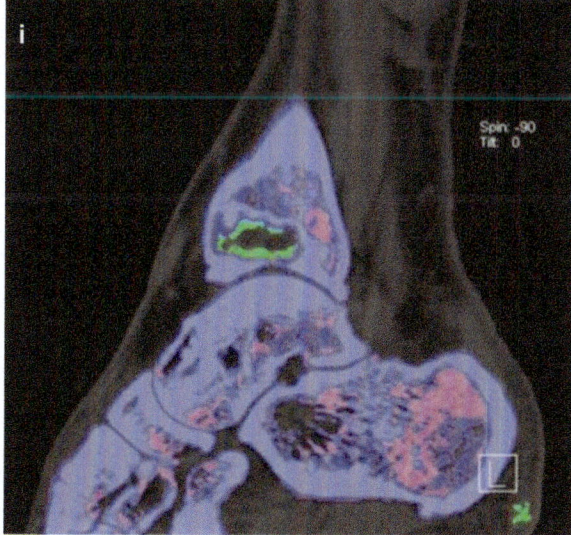

Fig. 9.1 (continued)

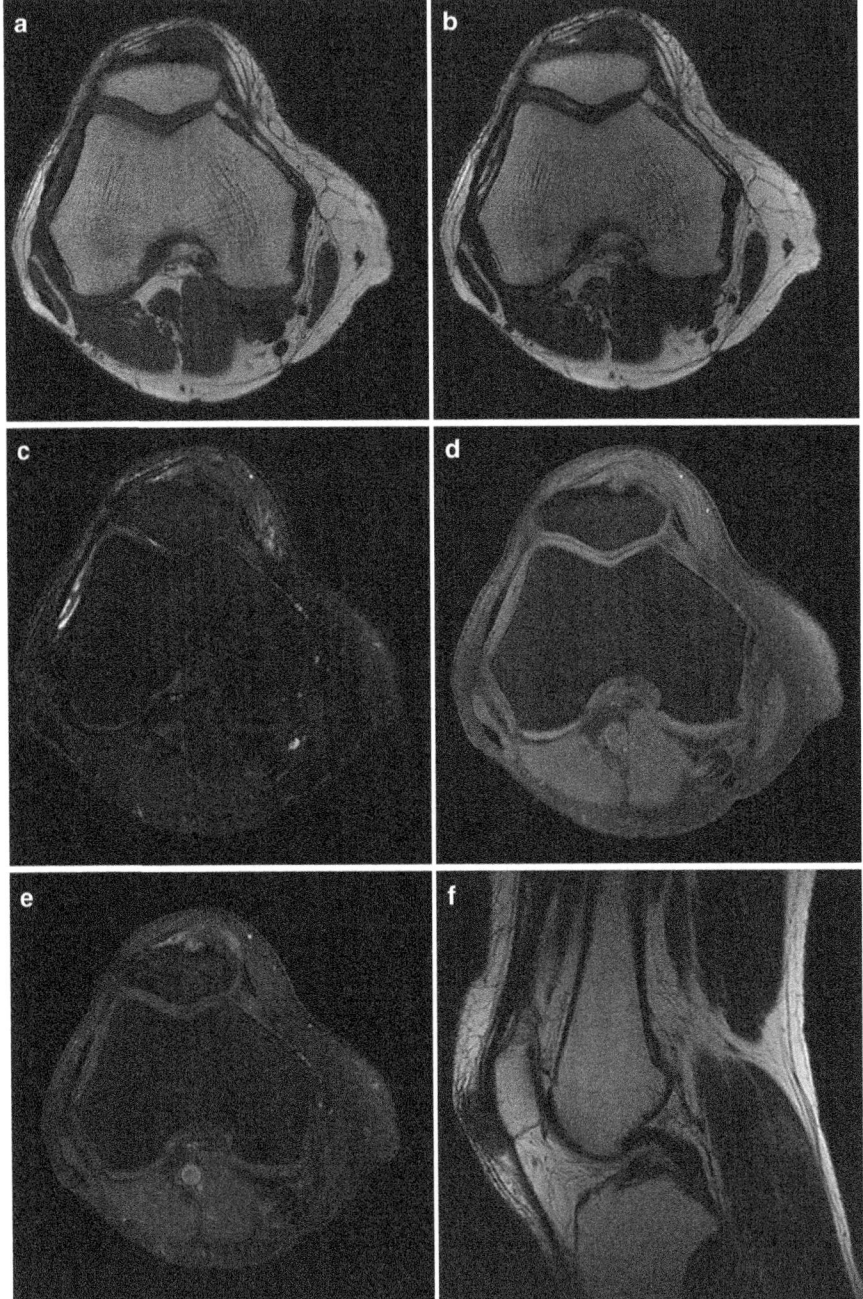

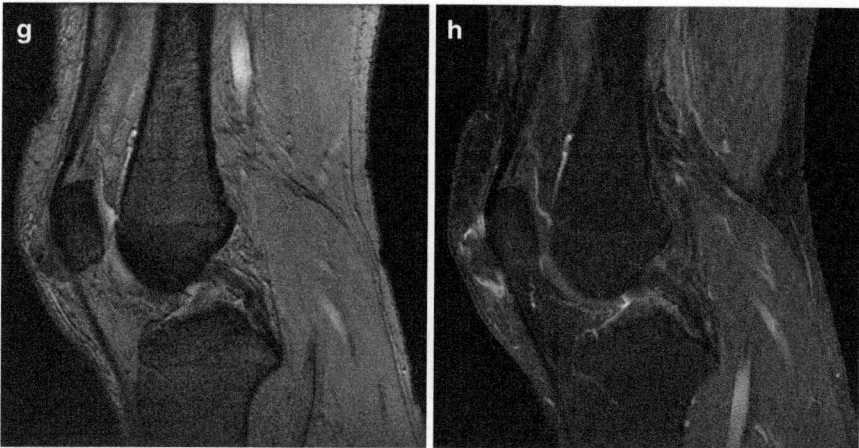

Fig. 9.2 (continued)

9.2.2   Pigmented Villonodular Synovitis (PVNS)

Benign synovial proliferative lesions are commonly encountered in musculoskeletal clinical practice. PVNS is an umbrella term that encompasses benign proliferative lesions involving the synovium of the joint, bursa, and tendon sheath. PVNS can present as a diffuse intraarticular, localized intraarticular, or localized extraarticular mass [2, 30, 32].

Synovial biopsy and histopathology provide the definitive diagnosis of PVNS [2, 30, 32]. Synovial proliferation with scattered multinucleate giant cells, macrophages, fibroblasts, xanthoma cells, and variable amounts of hemosiderin are present. Hemosiderin is helpful, but not a prerequisite for histological diagnosis [2].

Fig. 9.2 A 54-year old man presented with a growing lump in the anterior aspect of the right knee without history of injury. Axial T1 (**a**), axial T2 (**b**), axial fat-saturated T2 (**c**), axial fat-saturated T1 before (**d**) and after (**e**) administration of intravenous gadolinium, sagittal T2 (**f**), sagittal fat-saturated T1 (**g**), sagittal MPGR (**h**) MRI sequences demonstrated a 2.7 cm (transverse) ×1.3 cm (anteroposterior) ×2.5 cm (craniocaudal) subcutaneous mass that erodes into the anterior cortex of the patella. The mass demonstrates hypointense signal on T1, intermediate signal on T2, and heterogeneous enhancement without significant blooming on gradient-echo sequence. The MRI features of the mass are nonspecific, with broad differential diagnoses that include gouty tophus and a soft tissue sarcoma. We recommended dual energy CT

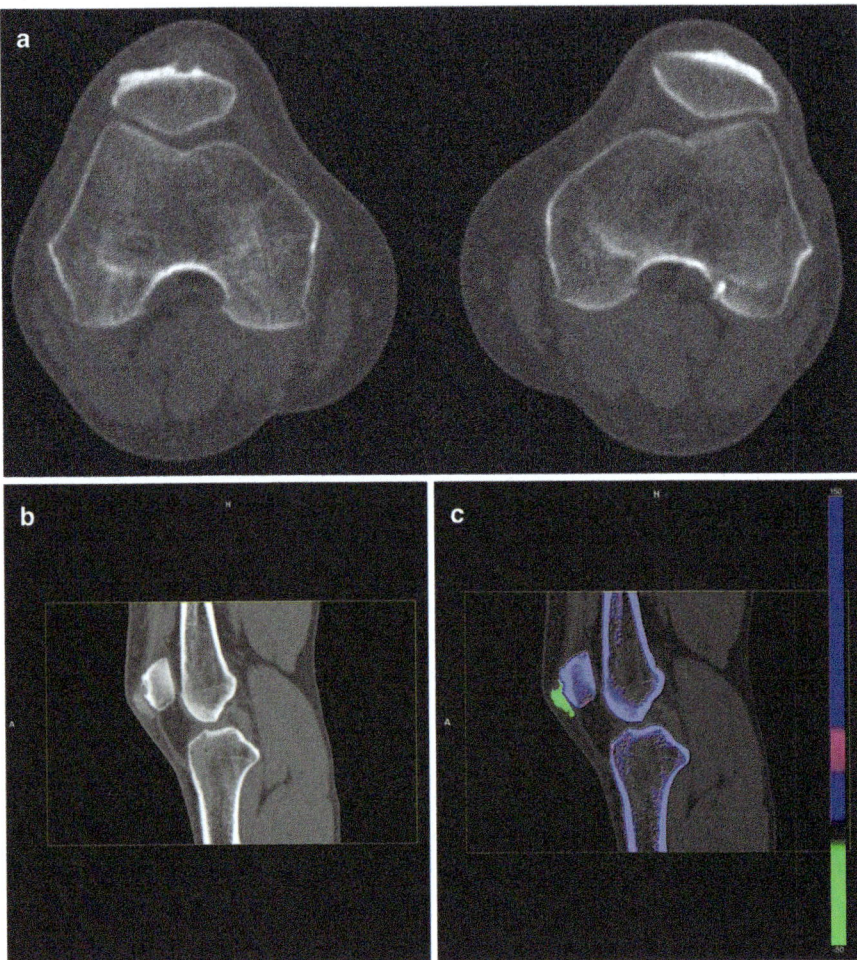

Fig. 9.3 Axial CT images of bilateral knees (**a**) and sagittal CT images of the right knee (**b**) show a mineralized right prepatellar mass with associated erosion of the anterior cortex of the patella Sagittal (**c**) sagittal reformatted image with DECT characterization confirms the mineralization as monosodium urate deposits (color coded as *green*), which is composed of C, H, N, and O are present within the prepatellar mass. Calcium, a heavy, high atomic number element with high attenuation of the low kV beam is color coded as blue. Trabecular bone is color coded as pink, (**d**) 3-dimensional volume-rendered coronal reformatted DECT of the right knee (R) shows the prepatellar tophaceous gout and the nonaffected left knee

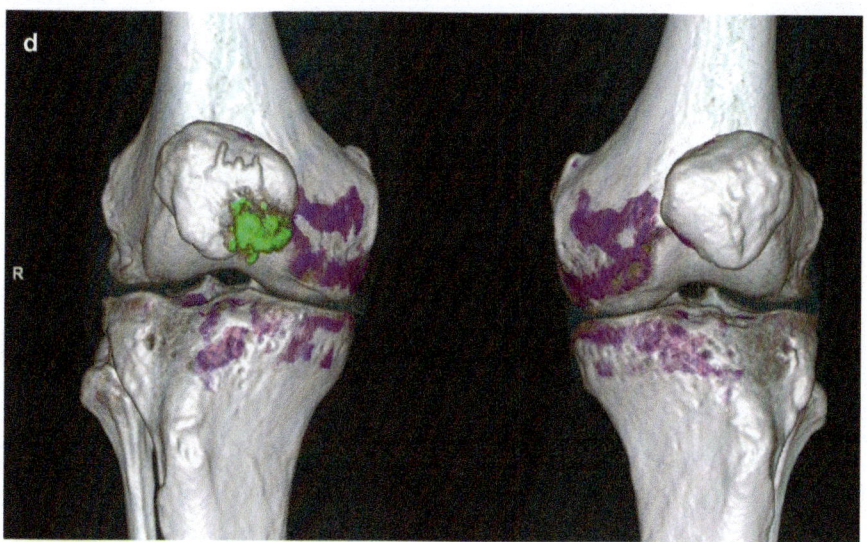

Fig. 9.3 (continued)

Furthermore, the extent of hemosiderin deposition is variable. Hemosiderin is usually a much more prominent feature of diffuse intraarticular PVNS [2]. Consequently,
we will focus on the diffuse intraarticular form of PVNS for the remainder of this
section.

The histopathology of the diffuse intraarticular form of PVNS can appear similar
to an aggressive sarcoma such as synovial sarcoma, rhabdomyosarcoma, and epi-
theloid sarcoma. These features include an extremely large cell size, invagination of
the cytoplasm into the nucleus (which resembles large nucleoli), and an increased
number of mitoses [2, 36, 38]. There is a large disparity in prognosis and treatment
between PVNS and sarcoma. PVNS can be treated with synovectomy, however,
sarcomas require removal of the tumor with clear margins, occasionally necessitat-
ing limb amputation [2, 36, 38]. Correlation of the histological features of the tissue
biopsy with the imaging findings of a diffuse synovial process plays an important
role in guiding the pathologist to the correct diagnosis.

MRI is the best imaging modality to detect this condition, due to the presence of
hemosiderin in these lesions [1, 2]. On T2-weighted images, low signal intensity
predominates due to preferential shortening of the T2 relaxation time caused by
hemosiderin. Gradient-echo sequence significantly accentuates this effect, resulting
in enlargement of the low signal intensity areas known as "blooming" [2, 3]. The
blooming effect is considered to be nearly pathognomonic of PVNS, although synovial hemangioma and hemophiliac arthropathy can give similar findings due to
intraarticular hemorrhage and synovial hemosiderin deposition [3, 4, 6, 7].

CT demonstrates synovial thickening and extrinsic erosion of bone on both sides
of the joint in diffuse intraarticular PVNS. CT scans without contrast may show

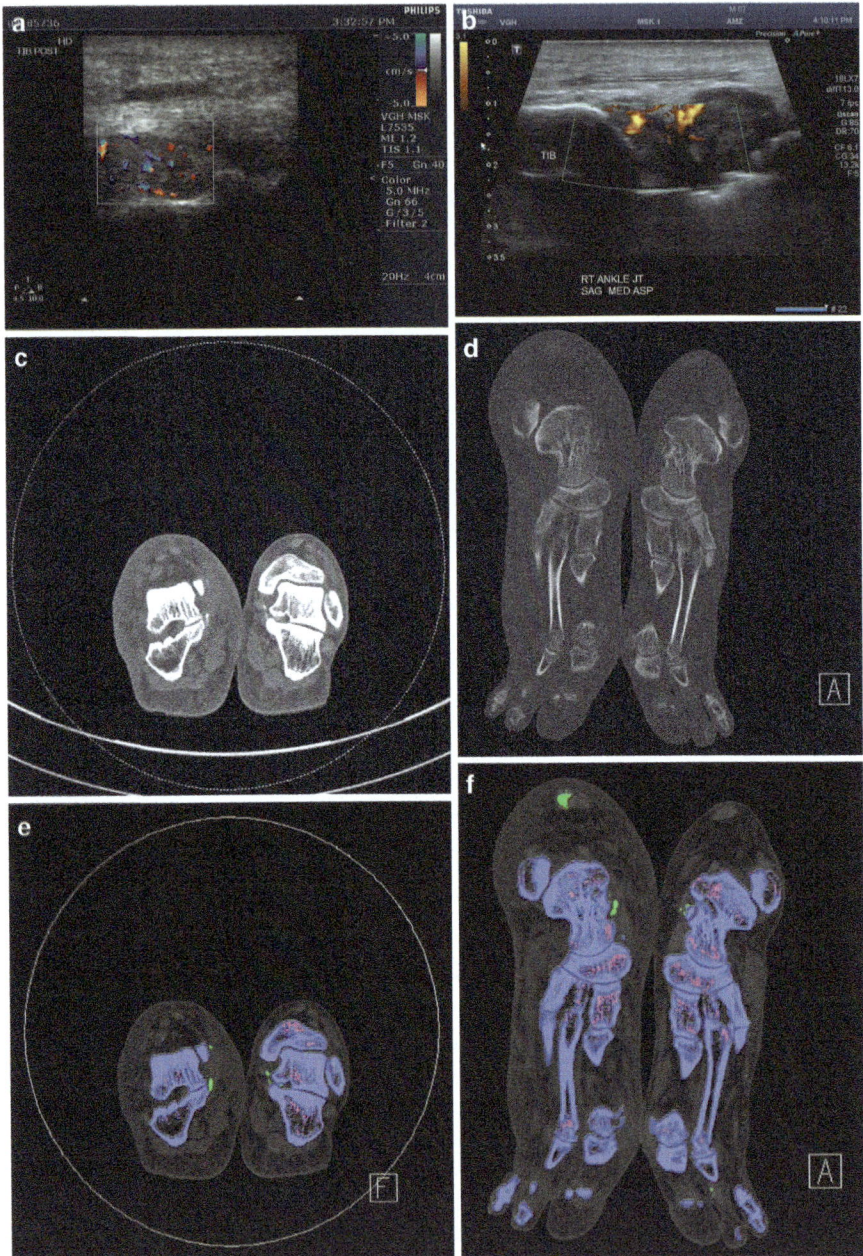

Fig. 9.4 (continued)

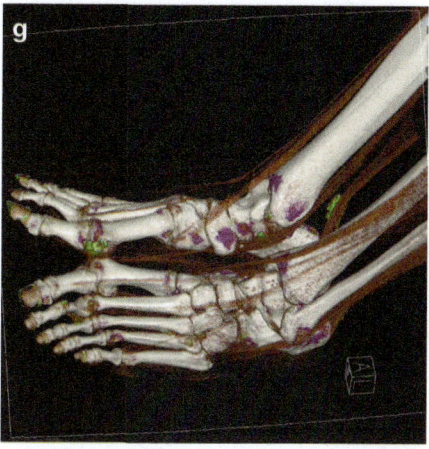

increased attenuation coefficient relative to that of muscle, due to hemosiderin content in the soft tissues [2, 8]. However, increased density is nonspecific and may reflect increased attenuation of other metals such as silicon, amyloid, copper, hemorrhage, calcium, or MSU crystals.

DECT has been utilized in the assessment of iron deposition within the liver; however, to our knowledge, there has been no published study on the use of DECT for detecting hemosiderin in soft tissue or bone lesions [8, 9, 11, 12].

9.2.2.1 "Hemosiderin/Iron" Application

The Liver VNC application enables the visualization of iodine contrast medium concentration in the liver without an additional noncontrast scan, even in the

Fig. 9.4 A 57-year old man with history of ulcerative colitis, hypertension, and gout presented with a mass that arises from the medial aspect of the right foot. (**a**, **b**) Ultrasound demonstrated a hyperemic 1.7 cm mass inferior to the medial malleolus that is contiguous with the medial aspect of the subtalar joint and deep to the tibialis posterior tendon. (**c**) Coronal and (**d**) axial CT images showed mineralization in this mass, associated with mild erosion involving the juxta-articular aspect of the medial subtalar joint. Note is made of mineralization in a similar area on the contralateral left foot and mineralization in a right Achilles peritendinous mass. After DECT analysis, coronal (**e**), axial (**f**), and 3-D volume-rendered (**g**) images confirmed mineralization as monosodium urate deposits. 3-D volume-rendered DECT images of both feet demonstrate the presence of monosodium urate within the peritendinous mass contiguous with the right tibialis posterior tendon, and deposits elsewhere in both feet including a peritendinous mass associated with the right Achilles tendon

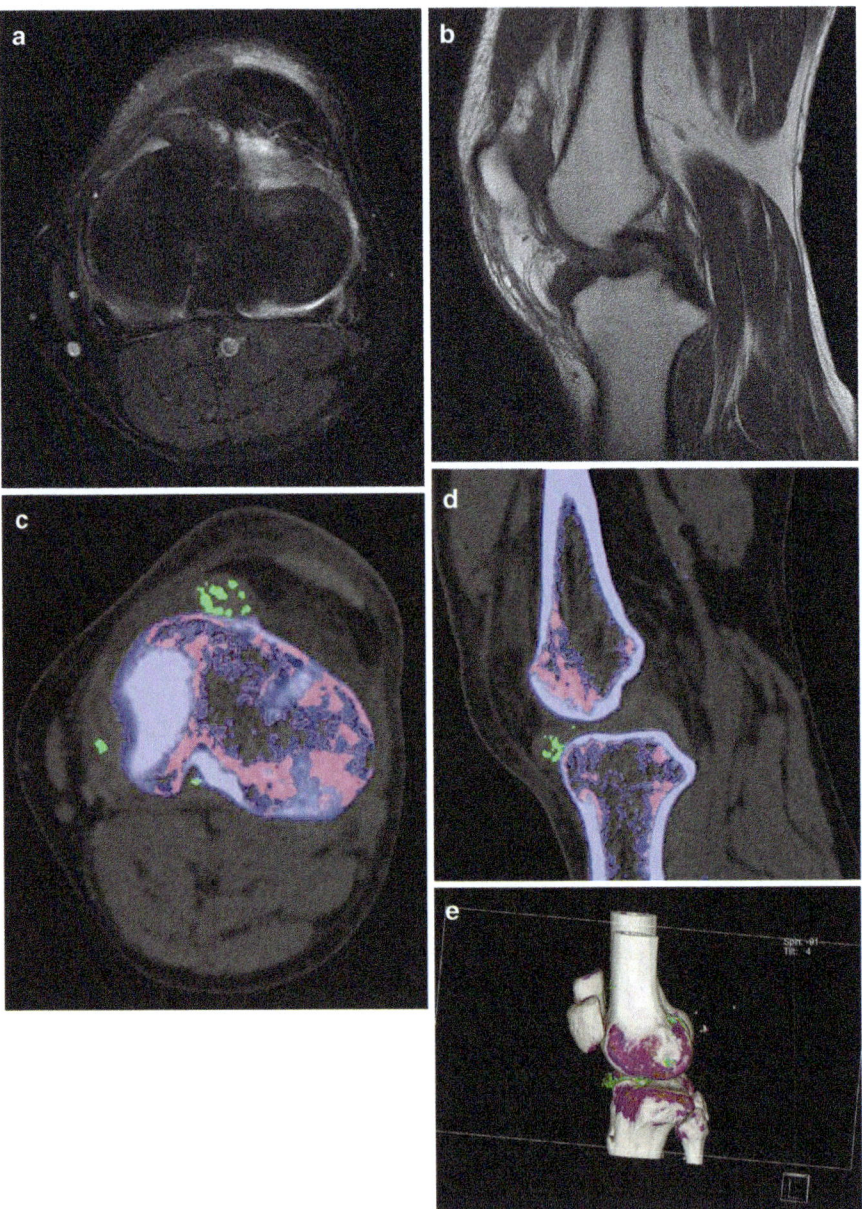

Fig. 9.5 A 55-year old man presented with left anterior knee pain. (**a**) Axial fat saturated PD FSE and (**b**) sagittal T1 FSE MRI images demonstrate an intra-articular mass contiguous with the anterior horn of the medial meniscus that is low signal on T1, T2, and fat saturated PD sequences, with a working diagnosis of pigmented villonodular synovitis. DECT axial (**c**), sagittal (**d**), and (**e**) 3-D volume-rendered images demonstrate monosodium urate within the intraarticular mass

Fig. 9.6 Based on a modified Liver VNC application where hemosiderin or iron has replaced iodine, the Syngo Siemens Dual Energy software tool demonstrates three-material decomposition of fat, soft tissue, and iodine/hemosiderin

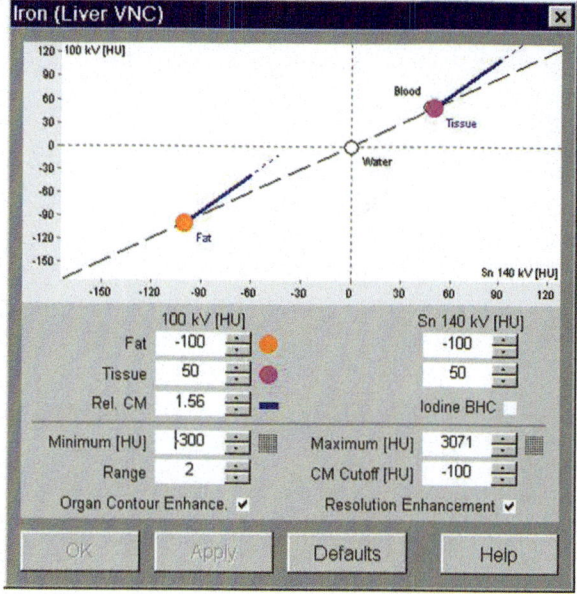

presence of irregular fatty infiltration of the liver or necrotic areas. The basis for this approach is a three-material decomposition algorithm with the three components being iodine contrast medium, fat, and soft tissue [11, 14].

For the purpose of detecting iron in a biopsy-proven diffuse intraarticular PVNS involving the hip, we modified the parameters in the Liver VNC application, by substituting iron/hemosiderin for iodine. Figure 9.6 demonstrates the altered key parameters. "Rel. CM," the parameter that contains the ratio of relative change in attenuation at 80 kV/100 kV and 140 kV for the material in question, in this case being iron/hemosiderin, is changed from 2.24 (which was for iodine) to 1.56 at 100 and 140 kV. "Fat," the parameter that contains typical HU-values of body fat, is altered to -100 for both 80 kV AND 140 kV. "Tissue," the parameter that contains typical HU-values of soft tissue, is changed to 50 HU for both 80 kV and 140 kV. Iodine BHC, which activates beam-hardening correction for iodine contrast enhancement and allows clearer visualization of calcified plaques and stents, is switched off because the material in question is hemosiderin/iron and no longer iodine.

9.2.3   Assessment of Vascular Masses

9.2.3.1 Body Bone Removal Application
The large attenuation differentiation between iodine (vascular component) and adjacent bone at low-energy levels allows us, with one sequential acquisition, to better delineate bone from adjacent vessels with one click utilizing the Syngo Via

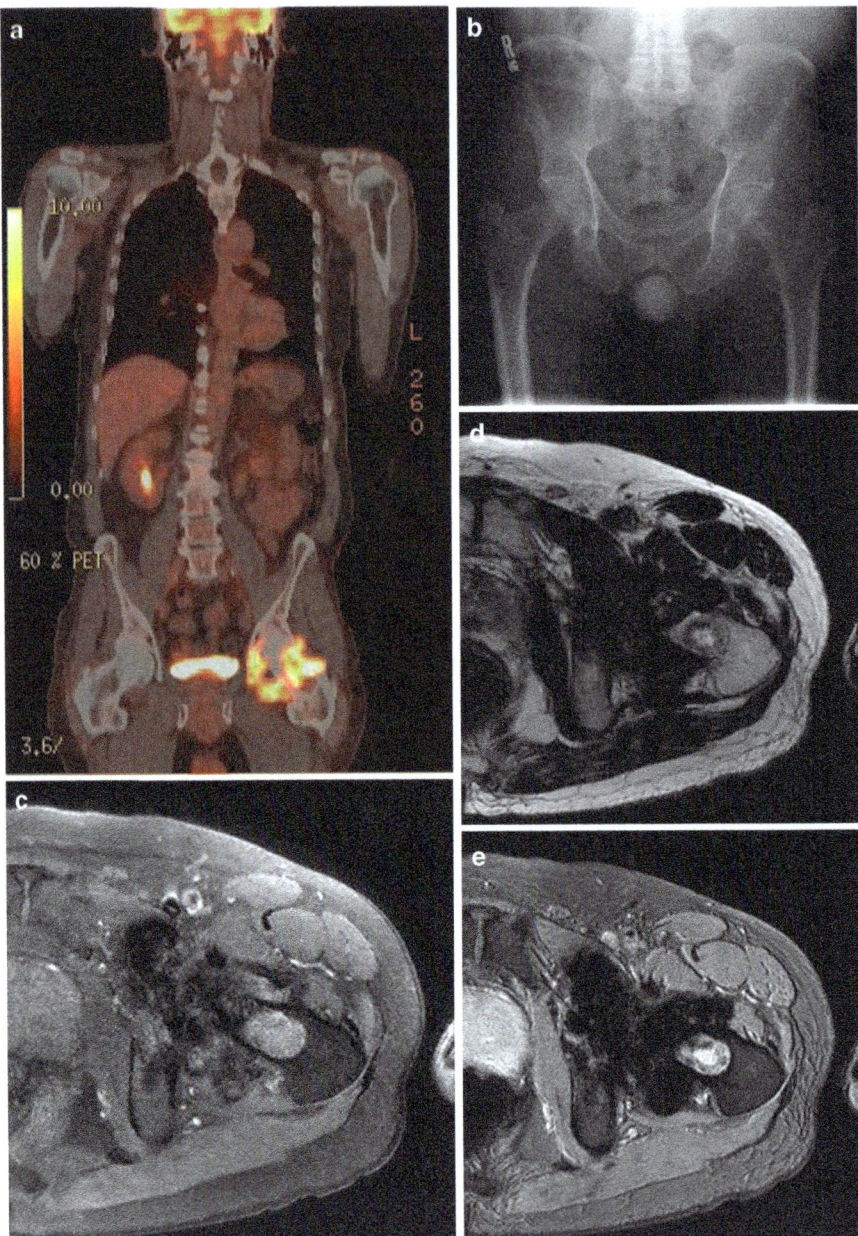

Fig. 9.7 A 66-year old man with squamous cell carcinoma involving the left base of tongue had a (**a**) staging PET scan that revealed diffuse and avid uptake in the left hip. Clinical examination revealed an irritable left hip. (**b**) Plain pelvic radiograph shows well-defined erosions in the left femoral head and neck. (**c**) Axial fat suppressed T1, (**d**) axial T2, (**e**) axial gradient echo, (**f**) coronal T1, and (**g**) coronal STIR images of the left hip demonstrate femoral erosions, synovial thickening with low signal intensity on T1 and T2 weighted images with "blooming" on gradient-echo images. DECT axial (**h**) and coronal (**i**) images demonstrate hemosiderin deposit (color-coded as *green*) in the medial aspect of the left hip joint space that correlates with the "blooming" hypointensities seen on MRI. Assigning different color coding for the hemosiderin deposits (**j**) can make the lesion more conspicuous

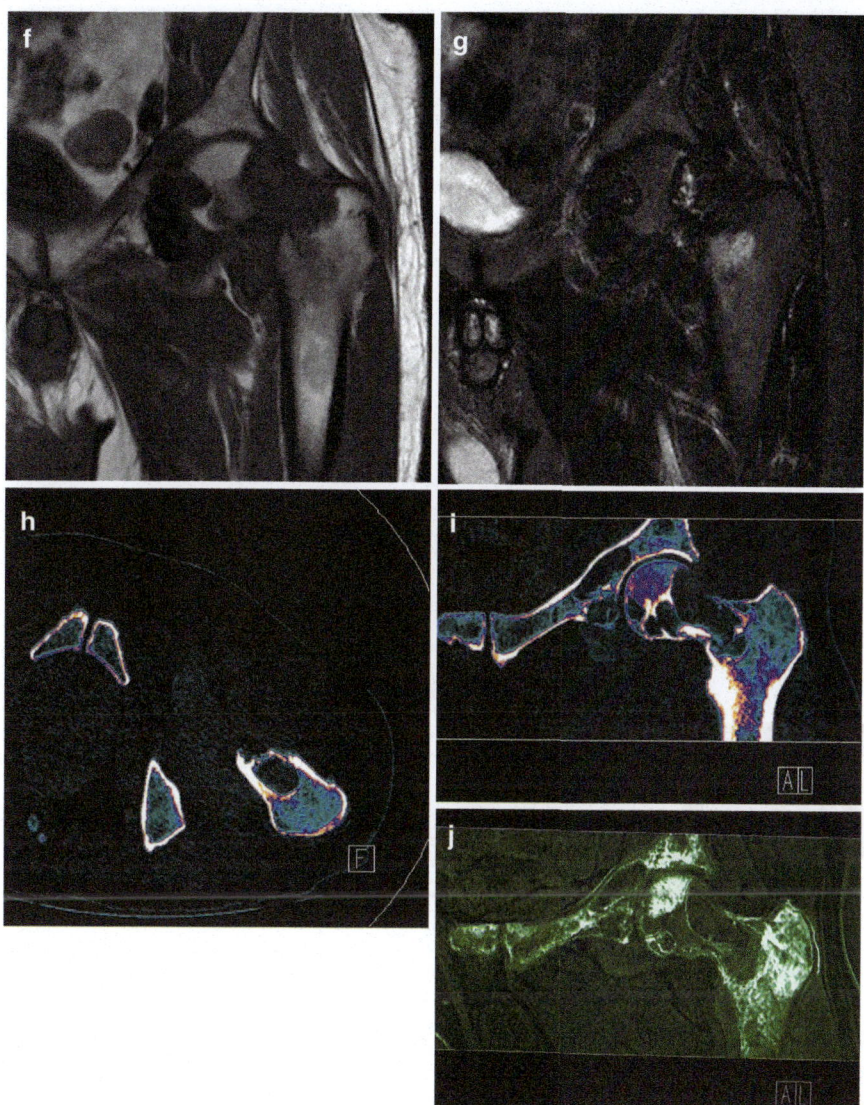

Fig. 9.7 (continued)

DECT vascular application. This is a faster and more accurate method than single energy techniques that require the need for a noncontrast scan and bone/vessel motion registration software [45]. This improves visualization of vascular tumors and provides better delineation of the vascular supply of the lesion using dual energy techniques. This also reduces onerous demand placed on technicians in postprocessing and reformatting the images to send to the PACS archival system (Fig. 9.8c).

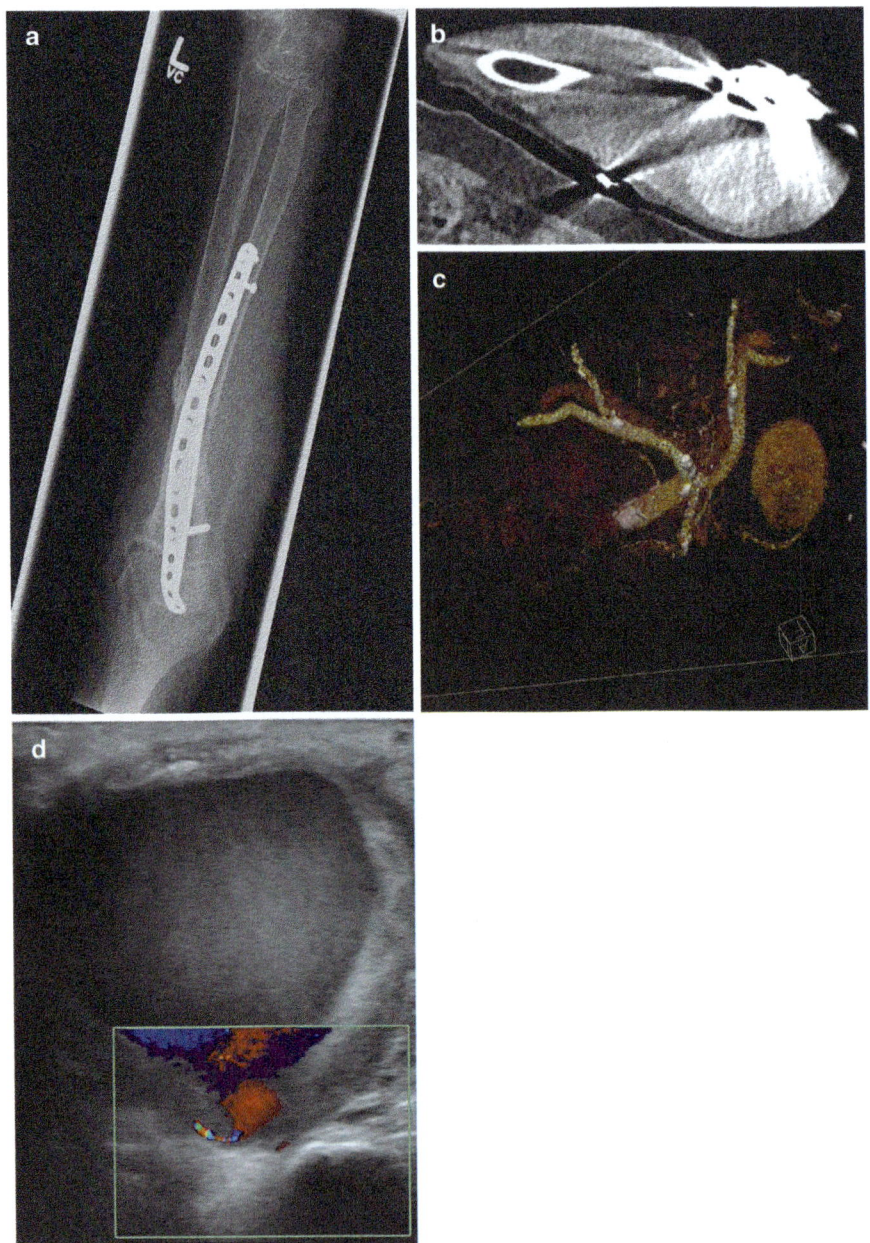

9.2.3.2 "Iodine Overlay" Liver VNC Application

Assessment of the relative vascularity of masses can be accurately assessed through tissue enhancement and iodine concentration on iodine maps. The distribution of iodine correlates with local perfused blood volume and vascular density, thereby assessing for angiogenesis and possible degree of malignancy in soft tissue masses. This allows for assessment of the mass as being benign or malignant or a surrogate biomarker for assessing treatment response [8, 14, 18, 19]. Iodine may increase the depiction and characterization of hypoattenuating lesions through an increase in the contrast between the lesion and the normal adjacent parenchyma on the basis of differences in tissue iodine content [11, 14, 18].

The relatively high atomic weight number and relatively high K-edge (33.2 keV) of iodine result in large changes in attenuation when two different x-ray energies are used to image the lesion in comparison to water, fat, and soft tissue [11, 14]. At the low kV spectrum, the photoelectric effect dominates as previously described. The attenuation of iodine increases exponentially as we approach closer to the k edge of iodine at the low kV energies of 70 and 80 kV. Given this principle, through dedicated post processing algorithms we not only can measure and segment iodine content but can also completely subtract iodine from adjacent soft tissue [6, 9, 25, 46]. Subtracting out iodine allows the creation of virtual noncontrast (VNC) images, thereby eliminating the need for a noncontrast acquisition. This reduces radiation exposure for the patient, while at the same time allowing for assessment of masses with a single scan [23, 24]. This is achieved via three-material decomposition in image space using modeled absorption characteristics of three materials. The concentration of iodine within the imaged vascular structures and masses can be quantified in milligrams of iodine per milliliter of tissue (Fig. 9.9a) or superimposed as an

---

Fig. 9.8 A 80-year female presented with an enlarging mass in the left forearm after open reduction and internal fixation (ORIF) of proximal to mid ulnar fracture (**a**) and sensory deficit consistent with ulnar nerve distribution involving the fifth digit. (**b**) Axial oblique DECT post intravenous contrast showed an enhancing ovoid mass that lies medial to the ulnar plate and screws. Monoenergetic function was used to reduce streak artifacts, allowing easy visualization of the mass. (**c**) 3-D surface-rendered DECT images after application of bone body removal application demonstrate the vascular anatomy of the mass. The mass is continuous with the proximal ulnar artery, possibly an interosseous branch of the ulnar artery. (**d**) Ultrasound demonstrated a complex cystic mass with highly mobile internal echoes adjacent to the proximal right ulnar artery. Color doppler showed swirling pattern of flow consistent with a pseudoaneurysm, most likely iatrogenic and related to prior ORIF of the midulnar fracture

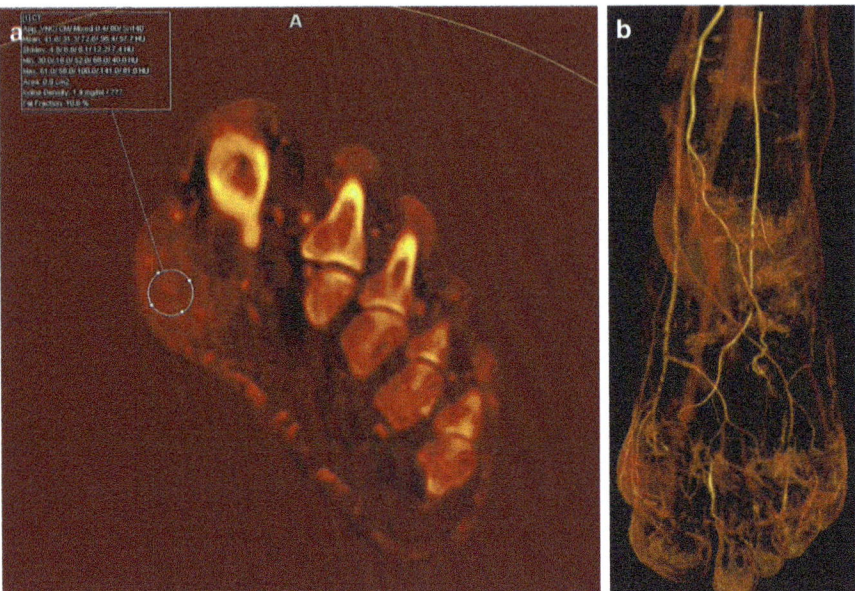

Fig. 9.9 A 77-year old man presents with a lesion at the planter aspect of the first metatarsopha-langeal joint of the left foot, which is not painful and slowly increasing in size. The Liver VNC application allows (**a**) the measurement of iodine within the mass and (**b**) an iodine overlay map or volume rendering (VRT) images that demonstrate the vascularity of the mass

overlay color "iodine map" that only depicts regions of iodine uptake (Fig. 9.9b) [11, 25]. The ability to quantify and map iodine distribution and create VNC images using DECT for musculoskeletal tumors may add depth and insight over routine conventional characterization of soft tissue and bony masses (Fig. 9.10).

9.2.4 Monoenergetic Functionality

The monoenergetic application calculates images that are equivalent to images acquired with a monoenergetic X-ray beam of a single selectable energy. This is achieved in image space by the extrapolation of the polychromatic DECT beams (80 and 140 kV) into single keV ranging from 40 to 190 keV. By adjusting the energy level of the image output, we can optimize the contrast between different materials by taking advantage of the magnitude of the different single energy levels.

DECT monoenergetic imaging can be utilized to improve tumor conspicuity in malignant hypervascular tumors [9, 26]. Image contrast at lower energies (80 kV) is significantly higher than at higher energies (140 kV) [11]. This has been demonstrated to be useful in the setting of early arterial enhancing lesions, such as HCC, hypervascularized metastases, and hypodense liver lesions in the abdomen [47–49]. The DECT technique works particularly well for compounds with large atomic

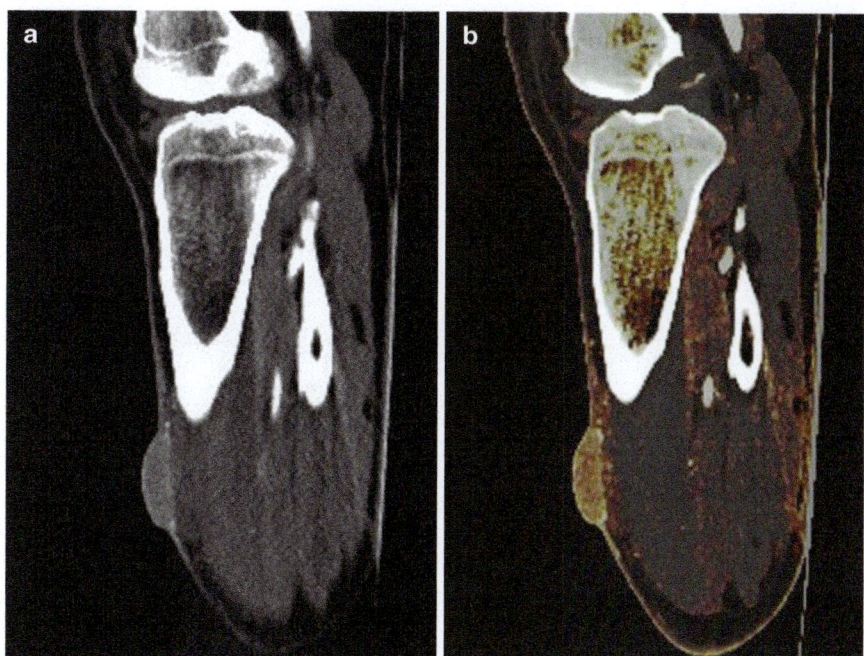

Fig. 9.10 A 73-year old man presented with a subcutaneous pretibial mass confirmed as on biopsy as a poroma, a benign skin tumor derived from sweat glands. The purpose of DECT was to assess for enhancement of the lesion and for involvement of underlying musculature or bone. Liver VNC application demonstrates avid enhancement within the solid portion of the mass and with expected background muscle and bone enhancement. We reported no evidence of involvement in the underlying tibialis anterior musculature or bony involvement. The mass was subsequently excised with clear margins and did not breach the deep fascia or extend into the underlying muscle or adjacent bone. Clicking the Mixed on/Off icon on the Application subtask card allows the user to switch between the (**a**) virtual non-contrast result volume and the (**b**) mixed CT volume

numbers by taking advantage of the photoelectric effect and the k-edge of iodine. Substances with higher molecular weight show exponential increases in attenuation behaviors at different energy levels [14, 17].

The use of low-energy images in oncologic CT imaging may improve lesion detection by improving contrast between a hypervascular lesion, a hypovascular lesion, and normally enhancing parenchyma [11]. Additional benefits of mooenergetic functionality, includes reduced image noise at higher kV values.

Hemosiderin deposits can be found in various soft tissue masses such as pigmented villonodular synovitis and giant cell tumor of bone [14, 17, 42]. Hemosiderin deposition, in theory, would allow for enhanced detection of various musculoskeletal soft tissue masses on DECT utilizing monoenergetic functionality. Pigmented villonodular synovitis has a higher image contrast at lower energies when compared with higher energies given its higher atomic weight compared to adjacent soft tissues depending on the concentration of iron within the soft tissues (Fig. 9.11).

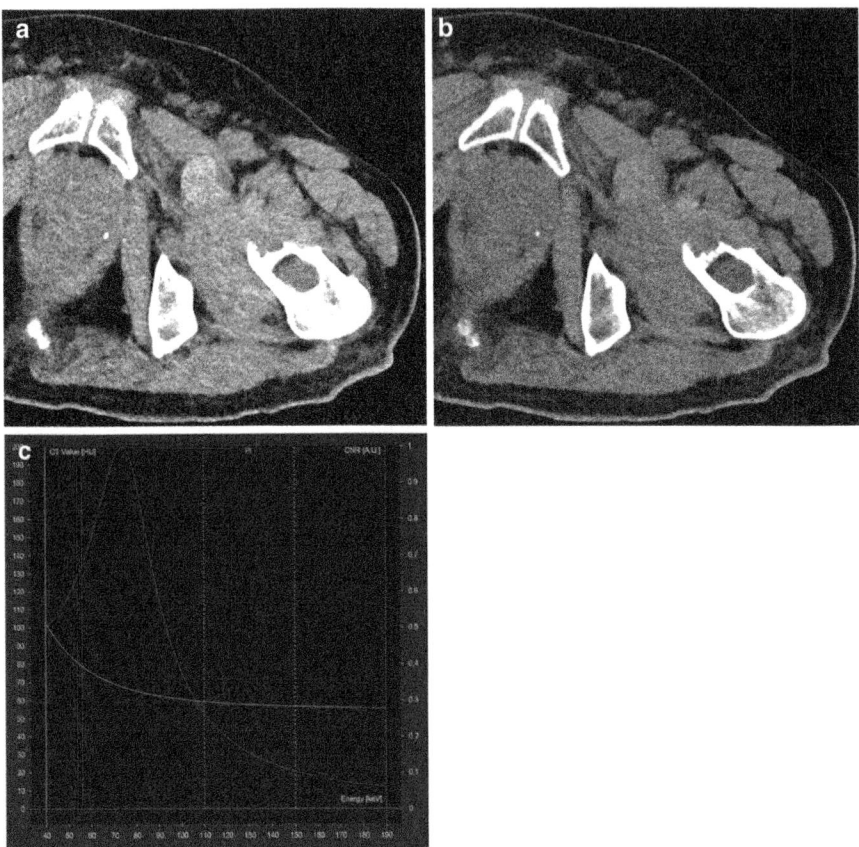

Fig. 9.11 Axial DECT images of the same patient in Fig. 9.7 shows (**a**) increased attenuation at low keV and (**b**) decreased attenuation at high keV. This is consistent with a high molecular weight compound, such as hemosiderin. (**c**) Spectral analysis curve of the same patient with PVNS. After drawing an elliptical region of interest (ROI) on the tissue of interest, clicking on the monoenergetic plus Spectral Information icon plots and calculates the estimated CT-attenuation value, iodine contrast to noise ratio versus photon energy, and slope of the curve for a region of interest. A diagram with two curves is displaced. The white curve (*left scale*) shows the calculated CT-attenuation value (HU) depending on the monoenergetic photon energy (keV). This curve differentiates between regions with different contrast media uptake. The blue curve (*right scale*) shows the calculated contrast to noise ratio (CNR) for iodine, depending on the energy level (keV). The curve is normalized to its maximum value. This curve optimizes the CNR for the present patient diameter and X-ray tube currents. In addition, the keV-region that is optimal for imaging of metal prostheses is indicated by the label "PI" and two *vertical dashed blue lines*

9.2.4.1 Spectral Curve Analysis

A useful function available within the monoenergetic application is the ability to display spectral information (Figs. 9.11c and 9.12). DECT has been shown to be useful in identifying properties of malignant transition areas, in particular microscopic invasion or simple bone marrow edema, by utilizing spectral curve analysis in malignant bone tumor intramedullary invasion in a rabbit model [50]. Analysis of the spectral curve was done by comparing the slopes of the spectral curves between 40 keV to 70 keV, as the slope is steepest within this range based on preliminary observations [50]. Through dual energy CT scanning, the polychromatic beams can be reconstructed between 40 and 190 keV, as previously described, which allows for the opportunity to detect subtle differences between two types of tissues. The generation of spectral curves from the DECT reflects the changes in CT attenuation values based on the elemental composition of tissues [51]. Different types of tissues have different types of spectral curves [52]. This produces characteristic fingerprints for different types of tumors based on their atomic weight composition. It is, therefore, feasible that similar principles apply to musculoskeletal soft tissue masses.

In the monoenergetic plus application, we can determine the energy value of the image output. The default value is 70 keV. Lower energy levels are useful for visualization of iodine and high atomic weight compounds. Higher energy levels are useful for visualization of soft tissues and low molecular weight compounds, as the attenuation of low molecular weight compounds increases mildly at the high kV levels [11, 14]. Literature has demonstrated that a wide spectrum of optimal monochromatic energies ranging from 95 to 150 keV can decrease beam-hardening artifacts and, thus, improve the image quality in the presence of metal prosthesis [53].

9.2.5 Bone Marrow Edema

The presence of hemorrhage and increased interstitial fluid within the bone marrow cavity characterizes bone marrow edema and results in small but measureable increases in CT attenuation values. Bone marrow edema is also associated with a wide variety of pathological processes including benign and malignant bone and soft tissue tumors [54]. MRI is sensitive for the detection of bone marrow edema as regions of low signal on T1 weighted sequence and high signal on T2 weighted sequence. This reflects the increase in fluid content of the marrow cavity. However, access to MRI can be limited and its use is contraindicated in some patients [55].

Detection of bone marrow edema utilizing conventional single energy computed tomography (SECT) has been attempted, and although attenuation based algorithms remove many bone structures, SECT methods are still unable to remove fine trabecular bone with sufficient quality to reliably reveal density changes in the bone marrow [55].

Given its relatively high atomic number ($Z=20$) and high dual energy index value, the calcium in trabecular bone can be successfully removed in DECT images using a process termed virtual noncalcium subtraction technique (VNCa) [56].

This technique subtracts calcium from cancellous bone, which allows better delineation and detection of bone marrow edema. This can be easily visualized with color-coded maps of the bone marrow edema and allows for more accurate quantification between normal and abnormal areas. We have found that virtual noncalcium subtraction can increase the conspicuity of bone tumors that are associated with bone marrow edema (Fig. 9.13).

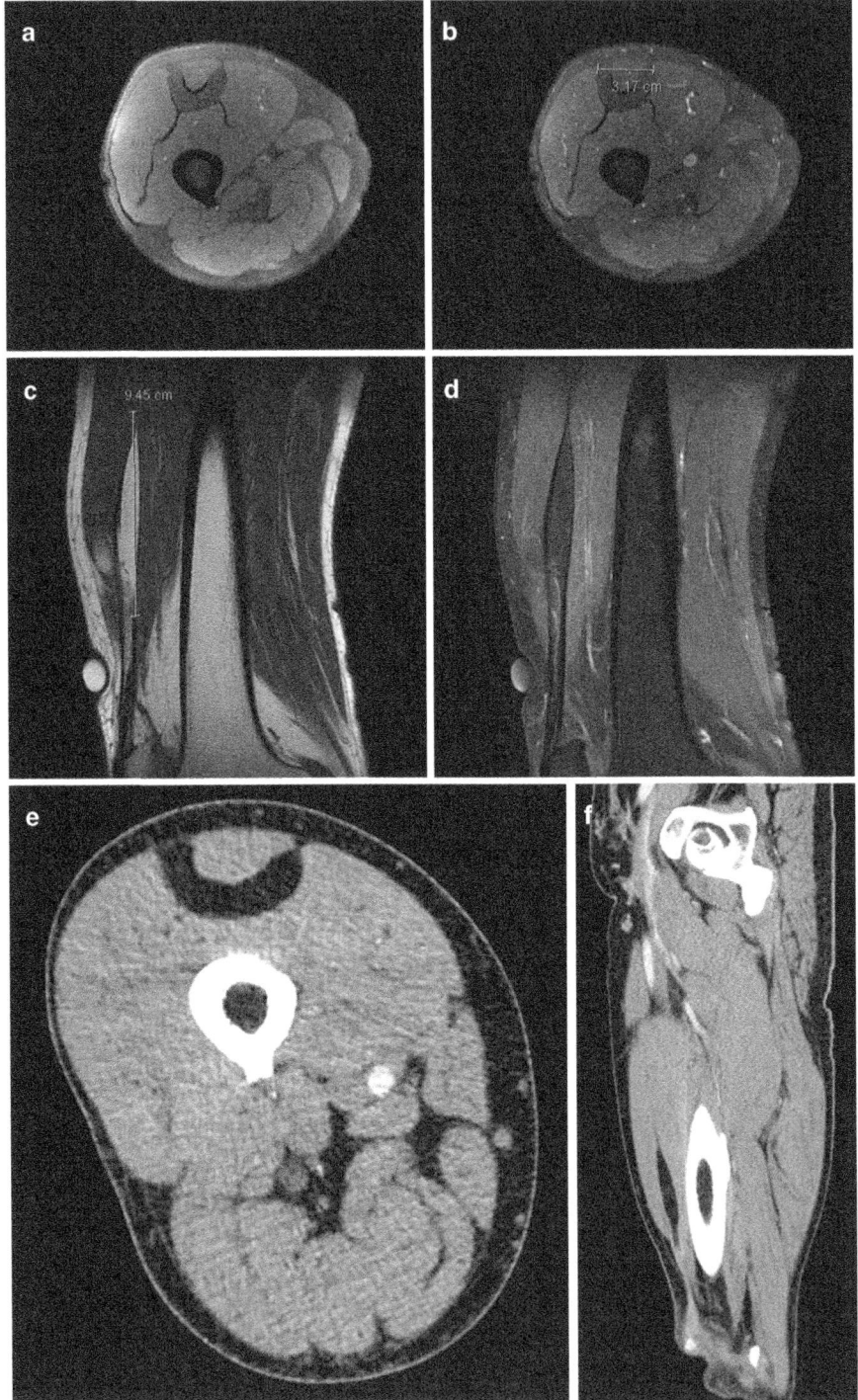

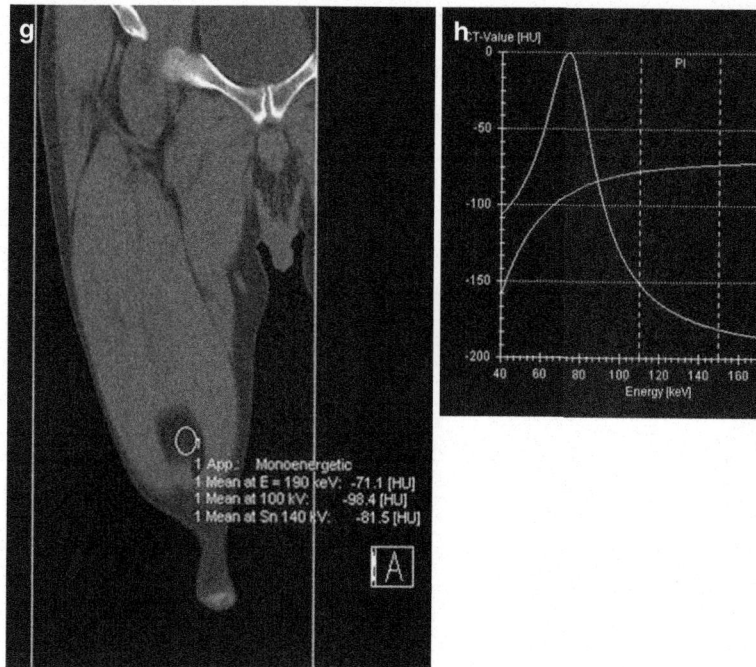

Fig. 9.12 (continued)

Fig. 9.12 A 58-year old male who presents with a right thigh mass for several months without pain or other symptoms. (**a**) Axial fat suppressed T1, (**b**) axial fat suppressed postintravenous gadolinium, (**c**) sagittal T1, and (**d**) sagittal fat-suppressed T1 postintravenous gadolinium images demonstrate an intermuscular fat containing mass posterior to the rectus femoris muscle that measures 9.5 cm in the craniocaudal direction, 1.3 cm anterior–posterior, and 3.2 cm in the transverse plane. This mass fully suppresses without evidence of soft tissue enhancement, consistent with a lipoma. DECT (**e**) axial, (**f**) sagittal, (**g**) coronal (with indicated region of interest), and (**h**) spectral analysis curve demonstrate a mass that demonstrates low attenuation at low keV and high attenuation at high keV, consistent with a low molecular weight compound such as fat. This mass was surgically removed and confirmed as a lipoma

9.3   Game Changer in Musculoskeletal Tumor Imaging

At our institution, DECT is increasingly being recognized by members of the musculoskeletal, bone, and soft tissue tumor group as a promising new and useful problem-solving tool in the work-up of soft tissue and bone tumors that presents from the entire province. DECT is unique amongst imaging modalities in its

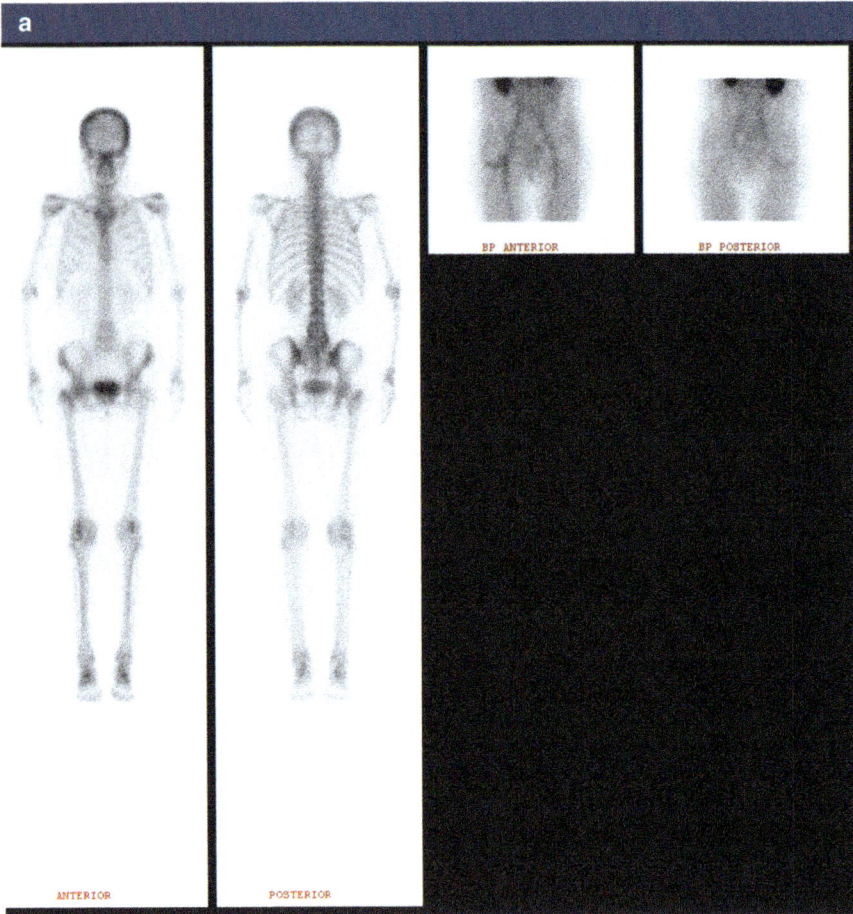

Fig. 9.13 A 66-year old female presents with pain in her right groin for 6 months. (**a**) Bone scan demonstrates mild increased uptake in the right femoral head and neck. MRI demonstrates a well-marginated lytic nonexpansile lesion in right femoral head and neck with preservation of primary compressile trabeculae that is (**b**) low on T1 and (**c**) high on T2 with mild reactive synovitis. (**d**) Virtual noncalcium-subtracted images and (**e**) corresponding color-coded three-material decomposition (calcium, water and fat) images show the presence of marrow edema which correlates to the low T1 and high T2 region on MRI. The imaging features of the lesion were consistent with an intraosseous hemangioma, which was confirmed with percutaneous biopsy

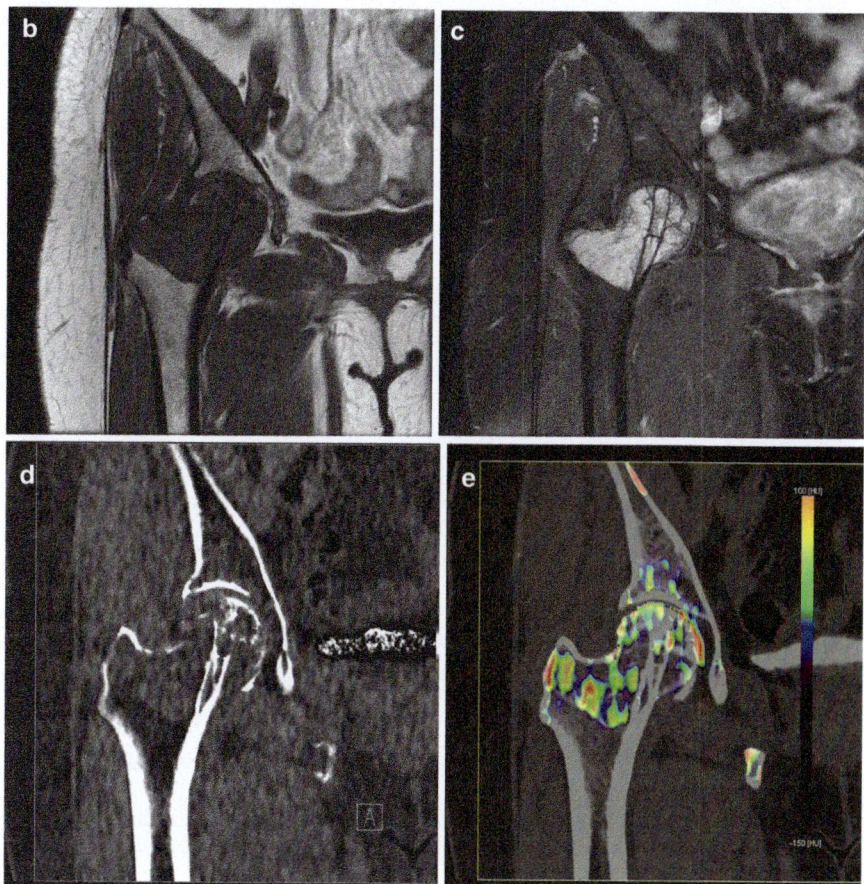

Fig. 9.13 (continued)

material differential capability in which patients are scanned with two distinct beam energies. In conventional CT imaging, materials with different chemical compositions can be represented by the same or very similar densities, making differentiation and classification of different types of tissues very challenging. DECT exploits the attenuation measurements acquired with different energy spectra and more importantly knowledge of the changes in attenuation between the two spectra to differentiate and classify tissue composition. This has significant implications for musculoskeletal tumor imaging. Despite the excellent ability of MRI to detect and characterize soft tissue and bone tumors, the majority of lesions remains nonspecific. The correct histological diagnosis reached on the basis of imaging studies alone is low, reportedly ranging from one quarter to one third of cases. DECT technology continues to evolve with future generation DECT scanners having the ability to scan at much lower and higher kV energy levels, which in turn allows for greater separation between low-energy and high-energy spectra with the use of more efficient detectors. The improvement in technology will allow more accurate characterization of the chemical composition of compounds. DECT has the potential to significantly improve the diagnostic specificity of musculoskeletal tumor imaging and be a game changer in our armamentarium of imaging techniques.

References

1. Zhu A, Lee D, Shim H (2011) Metabolic positron emission tomography imaging in cancer detection and therapy response. Semin Oncol 38:55–69
2. Murphey MD, Rhee JH, Lewis RB, Fanburg-Smith JC (2008) Pigmented villonodular synovitis: radiologic-pathologic correlation. Radiographics 28:1493–1518
3. Aksnes LH, Bauer H, Jebsen NL (2008) Limb-sparing surgery preserves more function than amputation a scandinavian sarcoma group study of 118 patients. J Bone Joint Surg Br 90:786–794
4. Rosenberg SA, Tepper J, Glatstein E et al (1982) The treatment of soft-tissue sarcomas of the extremities: prospective randomized evaluations of (1) limb-sparing surgery plus radiation therapy compared with amputation and (2) the role of adjuvant chemotherapy. Ann Surg 196:305–315
5. Malek F, Somerson JS, Mitchel S, Williams RP (2012) Does limb-salvage surgery offer patients better quality of life and functional capacity than amputation? Clin Orthop Relat Res 470:2000–2006
6. Nicolaou S, Liang T, Murphy DT et al (2012) Dual-energy CT: a promising new technique for assessment of the musculoskeletal system. AJR Am J Roentgenol 199:S78–S86
7. Dhanda S, Quek ST, Bathla G, Jagmohan P (2014) Intra-articular and peri-articular tumours and tumour mimics- what a clinician and onco-imaging radiologist should know. Malays J Med Sci 21:4–19
8. Chae EJ, Song J-W, Seo JB et al (2008) Clinical utility of dual-energy CT in the evaluation of solitary pulmonary nodules: initial experience. Radiology 249:671–681
9. Marin D, Nelson RC, Samei E et al (2009) Hypervascular liver tumors: low tube voltage, high tube current multidetector CT during late hepatic arterial phase for detection–initial clinical experience. Radiology 251:771–779
10. Simons D, Kachelriess M, Schlemmer H-P (2014) Recent developments of dual-energy CT in oncology. Eur Radiol 24:930–939
11. Agrawal MD, Pinho DF, Kulkarni NM et al (2014) Oncologic applications of dual-energy CT in the abdomen. Radiographics 34:589–612
12. Joe E, Kim SH, Lee KB et al (2012) Feasibility and accuracy of dual-source dual-energy CT for noninvasive determination of hepatic iron accumulation. Radiology 262:126–135
13. Cheng XG, You YH, Liu W et al (2004) MRI features of pigmented villonodular synovitis (PVNS). Clin Rheumatol 23:31–34
14. Johnson TRC, Krauss B, Sedlmair M et al (2007) Material differentiation by dual energy CT: initial experience. Eur Radiol 17:1510–1517
15. Dhanda S, Jagmohan P, Quek ST, Tian QS (2011) A re-look at an old disease: a multimodality review on gout. Clin Radiol 66:984–992
16. Garner HW, Ortiguera CJ, Nakhleh RE (2008) Pigmented villonodular synovitis. Radiographics 28:1519–1523
17. Remy-Jardin M, Faivre J-B, Pontana F et al (2014) Thoracic applications of dual energy. Semin Respir Crit Care Med 35:64–73
18. Hagspiel KD, Flors L, Housseini AM et al (2012) Pulmonary blood volume imaging with dual-energy computed tomography: spectrum of findings. Clin Radiol 67:69–77
19. Apfaltrer P, Meyer M, Meier C et al (2012) Contrast-enhanced dual-energy CT of gastrointestinal stromal tumors: is iodine-related attenuation a potential indicator of tumor response? Invest Radiol 47:65–70

20. Thiele RG, Schlesinger N (2007) Diagnosis of gout by ultrasound. Rheumatology (Oxford) 46:1116–1121
21. Lai KL, Chiu YM (2011) Role of ultrasonography in diagnosing gouty arthritis. J Med Ultrasound 19:7–13
22. Gerster JC, Landry M, Dufresne L, Meuwly JY (2002) Imaging of tophaceous gout: computed tomography provides specific images compared with magnetic resonance imaging and ultrasonography. Ann Rheum Dis 61:52–54
23. Sun C, Miao F, Wang X-M et al (2008) An initial qualitative study of dual-energy CT in the knee ligaments. Surg Radiol Anat 30:443–447
24. Jiang XY, Zhang SH, Xie QZ et al (2015) Evaluation of virtual noncontrast images obtained from dual-energy CTA for diagnosing subarachnoid hemorrhage. AJNR Am J Neuroradiol 198:840–845
25. Ho LM, Marin D, Neville AM et al (2012) Characterization of adrenal nodules with dual-energy CT: can virtual unenhanced attenuation values replace true unenhanced attenuation values? AJR Am J Roentgenol 198:840–845
26. Martillo MA, Nazzal L, Crittenden DB (2014) The crystallization of monosodium urate. Curr Rheumatol Rep 16:1–8
27. Bongartz T, Glazebrook KN, Kavros SJ et al (2014) Dual-energy CT for the diagnosis of gout: an accuracy and diagnostic yield study. Ann Rheum Dis 74(6):1072–1077
28. Dalbeth N, Pool B, Gamble GD, Smith T (2010) Cellular characterization of the gouty tophus: a quantitative analysis. Arthritis Rheum 62:1549–1556
29. Upadhyay N, Saifuddin A (2014) The radiographic and MRI features of gout referred as suspected soft tissue sarcoma: a review of the literature and findings from 27 cases. Skeletal Radiol 44:467–476
30. Vermesan D, Crisan D (2015) Synovial pathology. In: Prejbeanu R (ed) Atlas of knee arthroscopy, 1st edn. United Kingdom, London, pp 179–187
31. Roddy E, Choi HK (2014) Epidemiology of gout. Rheum Dis Clin North Am 40:155–175
32. Barile A, Sabatini M, Iannessi F et al (2004) Pigmented villonodular synovitis (PVNS) of the knee joint: magnetic resonance imaging (MRI) using standard and dynamic paramagnetic contrast media. Report of 52 cases surgically and histologically controlled. Radiol Med 107:356–366
33. Kuo C-F, Grainge MJ, Mallen C et al (2014) Rising burden of gout in the UK but continuing suboptimal management: a nationwide population study. Ann Rheum Dis 66:1374–1377
34. Hee LW, Singh VA, Jayalakshmi P (2010) Can gout mimic a soft tissue tumour? BMJ Case Rep. doi.10.1136/bcr.09.2009.2266
35. Li T-J, Lue K-H, Lin Z-I, Lu K-H (2006) Arthroscopic treatment for gouty tophi mimicking an intra-articular synovial tumor of the knee. Arthroscopy 22:910e1–910e3
36. Ferrone ML, Raut CP (2012) Modern surgical therapy: limb salvage and the role of amputation for extremity soft-tissue sarcomas. Surg Oncol Clin N Am 21:201–213
37. Amber H, Singh VA, Azura M (2012) Gouty tophi mimicking synovial sarcoma of the knee joint. Turk J Rheumatol 27:2006–2008
38. Nassar W, Bassiony AA, Elghazaly HA (2009) Treatment of diffuse pigmented villonodular synovitis of the knee with combined surgical and radiosynovectomy. HSS J 5:19–23
39. Du Y, Pullman-Mooar S, Schumacher HR (2005) Synovial sarcoma of the foot mimicking acute gouty arthritis. J Rheumatol 32:2006–2008
40. Sheldon PJ, Forrester DM, Learch TJ (2005) Imaging of intraarticular masses. Radiographics 25:105–119
41. Rettenbacher T, Ennemoser S, Weirich H et al (2008) Diagnostic imaging of gout: comparison of high-resolution US versus conventional X-ray. Eur Radiol 18:621–630
42. Deyle GD (2011) The role of MRI in musculoskeletal practice: a clinical perspective. J Man Manip Ther 19:152–161
43. Perez-Ruiz F, Dalbeth N, Urresola A (2009) Imaging of gout: findings and utility. Arthritis Res Ther 11:232
44. Melzer R, Pauli C, Treumann T, Krauss B (2014) Gout tophus detection-a comparison of dual-energy CT (DECT) and histology. Semin Arthritis Rheum 43:662–665

45. Schulz B, Kuehling K, Kromen W (2012) Automatic bone removal technique in whole-body dual-energy CT angiography: performance and image quality. AJR Am J Roentgenol 199:646–650
46. Heye T, Nelson RC, Ho LM et al (2012) Dual-energy CT applications in the abdomen. AJR Am J Roentgenol 199:S64–S70
47. Altenbernd J, Heusner TA, Ringelstein A et al (2011) Dual-energy-CT of hypervascular liver lesions in patients with HCC: investigation of image quality and sensitivity. Eur Radiol 21:738–743
48. Hur S, Lee JM, Kim SJ et al (2012) 80-kVp CT using iterative reconstruction in image space algorithm for the detection of hypervascular hepatocellular carcinoma: phantom and initial clinical experience. Korean J Radiol 13:152–164
49. Robinson E, Babb J, Chandarana H, Macari M (2010) Dual source dual energy MDCT: comparison of 80 kVp and weighted average 120 kVp data for conspicuity of hypo-vascular liver metastases. Invest Radiol 45:413–418
50. Chen H, Jia M, Xu W (2015) Malignant bone tumor intramedullary invasion: evaluation with dual-energy computed tomography in a rabbit model. J Comput Assist Tomogr 39:70–74
51. Coupal TM, Mallinson PI, McLaughlin P et al (2014) Peering through the glare: using dual-energy CT to overcome the problem of metal artifacts in bone radiology. Skeletal Radiol 43:567–575
52. Wang C-K, Tsai J-M, Chuang M-T et al (2013) Bone marrow edema in vertebral compression fractures: detection with dual-energy CT. Radiology 269:525–533
53. Bamberg F, Dierks A, Nikolaou K et al (2011) Metal artifact reduction by dual energy computed tomography using monoenergetic extrapolation. Eur Radiol 21:1424–1429
54. James SLJ, Panicek DM, Davies AM (2008) Bone marrow oedema associated with benign and malignant bone tumours. Eur J Radiol 67:11–21
55. Pache G, Krauss B, Strohm P et al (2010) Dual-energy CT virtual noncalcium technique: detecting posttraumatic bone marrow lesions–feasibility study. Radiology 256:617–624
56. Reagan AC, Mallinson PI, O'Connell T et al (2014) Dual-energy computed tomographic virtual noncalcium algorithm for detection of bone marrow edema in acute fractures: early experiences. J Comput Assist Tomogr 38:802–805

The manufacturer's authorised representative in the EU is Springer
Nature Customer Service Centre GmbH, Europaplatz 3, 69115 Heidelberg,
Germany. If you have any concerns regarding our products, please
contact ProductSafety@springernature.com

Printed and bound by CPI Group (UK) Ltd, Croydon, CR0 4YY
30/04/2026
02100659-0002